10 LAWS OF INSOMNIA

SOLVE THE PUZZLE OF POOR SLEEP AND
RECLAIM YOUR BEST LIFE

Robert N. Glidewell, PsyD, CBSM

The Insomnia Clinic™

ISBN-13: 978-1514102923
ISBN-10: 1514102927

Author photos by Teresa Lee (www.teresaleephotography.com)

http://www.coloradoinsomniaclinic.com

To all who long for a good night's sleep

CONTENTS

PART 5: BEYOND THE LAWS OF INSOMNIA

ACKNOWLEDGEMENTS

First and foremost, I owe profound thanks to my family. Without the tolerance and patience of my wife Katie, my parents, and my children Caitlin and Tucker, this book would not have been written. I love you all and thank God for the blessing of having you in my life.

I also wish to express overwhelming gratitude to my dear friend, colleague, and mentor William (Bill) Orr, PhD. While your professional encouragement and leadership have shaped my career, it is your friendship I most deeply value.

For inspiration, I owe thanks to my many patients, clients, and students over the years. You have taught me so much about courage, resilience, and humor in the face of adversity. Thank you for allowing me to do work I love and play a healing role in your lives.

I also wish to thank the countless friends and colleagues who have blessed me with their support and encouragement over the years. Gregory Ruff, MD, Timothy Rummel, MD, John Harrington, MD, James Kinsman, MD, Elizabeth Botts, PsyD, Emily Roby, PsyD, Richard O'Brien, MD, Robert Vogt, MD, Kenneth Lichstein PhD, Mary Delaney, PsyD, Brian DeSantis, PsyD, Teofilo Lee-Chiong, MD, Jeff Dyche, PhD, Michelle Beutz, MD, Jennifer Wink, MD, Gary Forrest, PhD, EdD, Franklin Willis, JD, Michelle Wine, PsyD, Brenda Mattson, Barbara Langerud, Natalie Marshall, Terry Jones, MD, Vandee Reyes, Jack Edinger, PhD, Bill Wenokor, MD, Ann Cartwright, PA, Corinne Andrews, Susan Cooper, PhD, Leilani Feliciano, PhD, Michele Okun, PhD, Kelly Orr, PhD, David Caster, MD.

Finally, I'm sure there is someone I've forgotten. I ask forgiveness of those who provided support and encouragement over the years and whose names I have failed to mention.

CHAPTER 1

INTRODUCTION

Bill entered my office and sat down in a blue chair. Well dressed and fit, in any other office he would be the most confident guy in the room. Not here. Not now. His confidence began to falter a few years before when a couple of bad nights of sleep during a business trip followed him home and turned into what he feared was a permanent nightmare.

At first it was only a couple of bad nights a week. He would feel poorly and avoid people and mentally challenging tasks on the following days. But...his inability to get a good night's sleep became more and more frequent and began to take its toll. He was quick to snap at his family and slow to respond at work. He didn't usually like to take medications and he certainly didn't believe in things like meditation and what he called "alternative mumbo jumbo." But we all do what we must when our back is against the wall.

By the time he came to sit in my office he had tried everything. Nothing had worked. He was afraid he was a hopeless case and he did not think anyone could help. He went on to say he was tired of spending money without results. He'd spent money and time on relaxation apps and acupuncture. He had hundreds of dollars' worth of pills and potions for sleep in his medicine cabinet. These just made him depressed when he opened the cabinet to see all of the money wasted for no benefit. Then he became very honest.

"Doc, I don't think you can help me either. At this point I think you're probably just another guy who wants to take my money but can't really make a difference for me. Another guy who wants me to spend more time and more money doing another thing that doesn't work."

This is how our conversation started. Fortunately, this wasn't the first time I'd come across this kind of doubt and mistrust. I told him what I tell almost everyone I work with in the beginning, "Well Bill, I don't know if I can help you but I want to understand your sleep story as deeply as I can. By the end of this conversation I'll let you know what I think is going on with your sleep, what can be done to fix it, and whether or not I feel like I'm the guy to help you do that."

After hearing his full sleep story I felt like I understood his sleep problem pretty well. He was a good fit for the insomnia clinic and the sleep transformation program. I saw him several more times and together we used the laws of insomnia I'm going to teach you in this book to bring about his personal sleep transformation.

Is this book for you?

This book is for people with insomnia, people who help people with insomnia, and people who love people with insomnia. Not sure if you have insomnia? No matter why it happens, if you have one or more of these problems several nights per week then you have insomnia:

- Does it take you more than 30 minutes to fall asleep? That's insomnia.

- Do you wake up more than once or twice per night? That's insomnia.

- Do you spend more than 30 minutes awake during the middle of the night? That's insomnia.

- Do you wake up early and can't get back to sleep many mornings? That's insomnia.

- Do you get plenty of sleep but never feel rested? That's insomnia.

- Do you have more than one of these problems? Now that's insomnia!

Still here? Then you must think you or someone you care about has insomnia. Now that we have that figured out, there are several reasons you will want to devour this book and move through it step by step.

You Want to Live Your Best Life

Being awake can be awesome, as long as you've had a good night's sleep. This book is going to talk a lot about how to overcome insomnia but that isn't really the point of the book. Ultimately the only reason you or anyone wants to read this book is because you want your life during the day to be as awesome as it possibly can be and poor sleep is keeping that from happening. The real reason to read this book is to reclaim your best life from insomnia, which has been dragging you down.

You Want a Cure, Not a Band-Aid

Using the basic laws of insomnia and the methods of sleep transformation I'll teach you in this book, you will literally reprogram your brain and body for healthy sleep. You can do this in a matter of weeks and the sleep transformation you achieve can last for years. This is because I'll teach you how to directly address the causes of insomnia, not just the symptoms.

You Want to Sleep Without a Pill

Have you ever talked with your healthcare provider about insomnia? If not, you're not alone. The average person with insomnia struggles for years before talking about it with their healthcare provider. Why is this? Most insomniacs don't want to have to take a pill to sleep and they know that's exactly what their provider is most likely to offer. In these pages you will learn exactly why most insomniacs don't need pills to sleep and how to go about building healthy natural sleep.

You're Tired of Spending Money Trying to Fix Insomnia

How much have you spent on your insomnia in the last six months? Twelve months? Five years? Do you feel it's been money well spent? You may be able to fix your insomnia for as little as the cost of this book. Keep reading and you may be able to set yourself free from paying for pills or other sleep solutions month after month.

You're Tired of Spending Time and Energy on Things That Don't Work

How happy are you with what you're doing for your sleep problem right now? Are you 100% satisfied with your sleep? 60% satisfied? 30% satisfied? Less? There is a solution to every sleep problem. If you are not at least 80% satisfied with your current sleep pattern, then whatever you're doing is not working. In these pages you will learn why you are probably one of the 90% of insomniacs who can take control of their insomnia without any special tools, pills, or potions.[1] You will also learn why you may be one of the 40% of insomniacs who can completely eliminate their insomnia without pills.[1]

You're Tired of Feeling Out of Control and Misunderstood

Do you feel as if your sleep is under the influence of some mysterious force you have no control over? Does someone you care about suffer from a sleep problem that makes no sense to you? I talk to people every week that are frustrated and confused how something as natural as sleep can be so out of control. In these pages you will learn how insomnia can take hold of anyone and why it makes us feel so crazy and disconnected.

You Want To Stop Taking Sleeping Pills

How long have you been taking sleep medication? How many have you tried? Have you tried to stop taking them only to find your insomnia worse than when you started? Many insomniacs who use the sleep transformation strategies I teach in this book find they can reduce or eliminate their use of sleeping pills. Why? Because when you effectively tackle the basic causes of insomnia you no longer need to mask the symptoms with medication.

Why should you trust me or what I have to say?

If you wanted to give yourself the best chance for transforming your sleep patterns and getting free of sleep medication, what would you do? Who would you trust to help you do that? If you want world-class help, then you want a specialist in what is called Behavioral Sleep Medicine - an insomnia expert with the most advanced training in sleep and the factors that cause almost every case of chronic insomnia. As I write this there are just over 200 clinicians in the world with this particular training, expertise, and experience.[2] I just happen to be one of them.

I've spent the majority of the last decade immersed in the spectacular world of sleep and sleep disorders in order to become an insomnia expert. From networking with some of the world's top scientists and thought leaders to publishing my own original research in family medicine and sleep medicine journals it has been quite a fascinating journey.[3-5] Because of this, I have a deep understanding of the research and when I teach these methods I'm not expressing opinion but teaching the most powerful strategies that I and the best scientists in the field have discovered and tested.

As one of a few clinical psychologists in the world recognized by the American Board of Sleep Medicine as a Certified Behavioral Sleep Medicine Specialist, I have had the unique privilege of spending thousands of hours helping people solve everything from the simplest of sleep problems to the most chronic and complex forms of insomnia. This experience means that I know how sleep works, I know how insomnia works and I know how to fix it. This is why I may just be the person to help you take control of insomnia and reclaim your best life through better sleep.

Why write a book about it?

This book is partially a product of frustration, even anger if I am truly honest, with the unfortunate realities of our healthcare system. A healthcare system that gives costly and risky medication treatment a privileged status over equally effective, less costly, and less risky alternatives that are readily available but rarely offered or even considered. As an example I want to tell you a story about Clubfoot.[6]

Children with Clubfoot are born with their feet turned inward and it can be crippling if not treated very young. Traditionally, treatment for Clubfoot involves repeated surgeries. These surgeries create a buildup of scar tissue that often leaves children with a lifetime of chronic pain, stiffness, arthritis and medical bills. Not good. Right?

Have you ever heard of Ignacio Ponseti? Unless you or a child in your family was born with clubfoot, probably not. The problem is that, until recently, the parents of children with clubfoot had never heard of him either. Dr. Ponseti was a physician at the University of Iowa. In the 1950's he developed a treatment for Clubfoot that uses a system of special leg braces that gradually normalize the child's legs and joints. It requires no surgeries, no pain, has similar outcomes, and leaves the child to walk normally through life without arthritis. This treatment is rarely offered however.

Why? In a 2014 interview Dr. John Herzenberg, then an orthopedic surgeon at Sinai Hospital in Baltimore, suggested, "Surgeons are trained to operate...and usually that's the way to make money. The Ponseti method brings in a lot less for orthopedists. So for about 50 years, the technique mostly stayed in Iowa." (To read a news story and see pictures, do a Google search for, "How Parents and the Internet Transformed Clubfoot Treatment.") So, for 50 years our healthcare system continued to perform surgeries on infants that left them with lifelong pain because of what?

8

I use this example because there is a similar situation with insomnia. Non-medication solutions for insomnia exist. They are cheaper than medication. They are as effective as medication. They are safer than medication. Patients prefer them over medication when they are offered. But they're not. For less than the cost of an office visit copay you could learn how to take control of your insomnia - without waiting for an appointment, without approval from your insurance company, and without side effects - but this has likely never been suggested.

UNACCEPTABLE.

Sleep is critically essential for maximum health and vibrant living. When you struggle to sleep, you should not have to fight to find a solution. I started the Sleep Health Revolution (See Chapter 3) and wrote this book to provide easy affordable access to proven sleep transformation strategies for people like you who struggle with insomnia and don't want a pill to sleep.

I also have a second and more personal reason for writing this book. There is a point in the process of helping a person with insomnia when I ask them to make changes that can be challenging, somewhat unpleasant, and often don't seem to make much sense. This is the point when, feeling both hopeful and apprehensive, they ask what may be the most important questions of the whole process, "Doc, how do you sleep? Have you ever had insomnia? Have you ever had to do the things you're asking me to do?"

I answer by telling them I do sleep well, even great, much of the time...as long as I follow my own advice. I answer by sharing my own insomnia story. That I would be considered to have what is called Idiopathic Insomnia, which is fancy medical speak for being born with a finicky sleep system that makes me particularly sensitive to things that disturb sleep. That on top of that, I am also a major night owl, a tendency that compounds my difficulties sleeping. Then I answer by telling them how I have gone through my own sleep transformation. That I have made the changes I am asking them to make. That I know only too well the apprehension and doubt as well as the sense of calm and confidence that come from making those changes (You can read more of my story in Chapter 2).

Ultimately, for many of those I work with, there seems to be reassurance in knowing that I have walked the very path I am asking them to walk, and come out the other end for the better; that I know deeply the struggle and the doubt, as well as the confidence that are part of the process. There is also reassurance in the fact that I have helped so many others walk this path, and they have a guide who knows the path so intimately.

Is there proof that sleep transformation actually works?

Some of you will be satisfied with the fact that I have not only made it through my own struggle with insomnia but also have helped hundreds of others find sleep transformation. Some of you will want more. If you are a person who wants some hard evidence that insomnia can be transformed quickly and without pills, you won't be disappointed. You can have reassurance that the path of sleep transformation has been rigorously tested and found both reliable and effective.

A search of the PubMed research database finds more than 100 studies, including numerous placebo controlled clinical trials, showing that what I call sleep transformation training (known in the research as Cognitive-Behavioral Therapy for Insomnia or CBT-I) is effective. In fact, the Journal of the American Medical Association (JAMA) published one of the most rigorous clinical trials comparing CBT-I to the sleep drug Ambien in 2009.[1] In this study, 90% of insomnia patients experienced clinically significant improvement and 40% experienced complete remission of insomnia symptoms. CBT-I was as effective as medication and, whereas long term medication use led to an increase in insomnia symptoms, participants who used CBT-I continued to experience growing improvements in their sleep up to a year after they stopped the treatment. Why is this? While sleep medications mask or cover up insomnia symptoms, CBT-I changes many of the actual causes responsible for almost every case of chronic insomnia.

This same body of research also shows that non-medication treatments can transform insomnia of years or decades in a matter of weeks. In fact, at the international sleep conference in Minneapolis in 2014, sleep researcher Colin Espie shared some amazing information.[7] When he and his team analyzed data from 1000 insomniacs who had participated in his online sleep transformation program they found that no matter how long they had insomnia, it got better. They also found that no matter how severe the insomnia was, it got better. This is the fact that most of the folks I work with respond to with the greatest skepticism. They struggle to believe that severe, long-standing insomnia can be transformed without pills in a matter of weeks. Of course, they are pleasantly surprised when the insomnia that has plagued them for years or decades begins to change course after only a few visits in The Insomnia Clinic.

If the couple of studies I shared above aren't enough to convince you, there is one last thing I would like to share. In 2005 when I was just getting started in the field of sleep and sleep disorders I had the privilege of attending what is called a State-of-the-Science conference hosted by the National Institutes of Health in Bethesda, Maryland. A State-of-the-Science conference is a meeting of top experts and scientists within a particular area of medicine who meet to determine exactly what is known and make recommendations to clinicians and scientists around the world. The conference in 2005 was on the management of chronic insomnia in adults. After reviewing the research at the time, they reached these conclusions about sleep transformation training:[8]

- It is as effective as prescription medication for treating chronic insomnia

- Its beneficial effects last well beyond the end of treatment

- There is no evidence that it produces any adverse effects

This was an exciting thing to witness as a young scientist and clinician. If I hadn't already decided to specialize in insomnia, seeing the science pointing in the direction that interested me in such a clear and powerful way would have pushed me over the edge. Imagine learning at the beginning of your career that there was something so powerful but relatively unknown and underused that could change lives so quickly.

What's special about this book?

The work we do at The Insomnia Clinic™ and the knowledge and techniques I'll teach you in this book are based on Guided Sleep Discovery™ and Radical Sleep Transformation™, two systems I've created to maximize your ability to eliminate insomnia without pills. These systems are based on what I call the "The 10 Laws of Insomnia."

The laws are fundamental principles that drive sleep and insomnia. Each law is based on brain and behavior research about how we create healthy sleep versus insomnia. When you understand these laws you can apply them to take control of insomnia and restore healthy natural sleep. If you follow these laws you will be changing your brain and body in a way that is proven to improve sleep in as many as 90% of those with insomnia.

Although some of the research underlying these laws has been around for more than 40 years, like Dr. Ponseti's treatment for club foot, the laws of insomnia have been largely ignored by traditional healthcare. This is why the most commonly offered treatment has been sleep medications. Unfortunately, any insomnia solution that ignores these laws is not actually a solution; it's just a Band-Aid covering up the symptoms.

How should I use this book?

The book is written to guide you through the process of Guided Sleep Discovery and Radical Sleep Transformation as you read through the chapters in order. However, you can also benefit from going to any chapter that seems most helpful or relevant to you. With that said, if you are doing the things I recommend and they are not working for you, don't give up. If my recommendations are not working for you then there is probably some part of your sleep puzzle that has not been figured out yet. I strongly encourage you to go back to the beginning and walk through the full process.

What's actually in this book?

Here's what you'll find in the rest of the book, chapter by chapter.

Chapter 2: Want to know more about my personal journey? I share my personal story of insomnia and sleep transformation and my experience of moving from insomniac to insomnia expert.

Chapter 3: I describe my experiences of frustration and disillusionment within our healthcare system that led me to create The Insomnia Clinic and start the Sleep Health Revolution.

Chapter 4: How has insomnia changed your life? You're not alone. This chapter looks at the way insomnia restricts health, performance, relationships, and happiness, and guides you in starting to tell your sleep story.

Chapter 5: Why do you have insomnia? When suffering from insomnia it can often seem like a mysterious force has control of your sleep and you are powerless to stop it. Fortunately, sleep is not a mystery. This chapter shows you the most common causes of insomnia and gets you started in the Guided Sleep Discovery process and solving your insomnia puzzle.

Chapter 6: What are your reasons for having insomnia? No matter what you have going on you can almost certainly sleep better. Insomnia has a life of its own and this chapter will give you the answer to why you should fight it no matter what.

Chapter 7: What are you doing to fix your insomnia? If it makes sense, it may be helping you survive but it's probably making your insomnia worse. This chapter shows you why you've been doing everything wrong, why trying to fix insomnia can be so frustrating, and why you shouldn't feel a bit bad about it.

Chapter 8: Ready to take control? Sleep power controls your ability to fall asleep, sleep deeply, and stay asleep. This chapter teaches you about sleep power and how you can quickly build up and manipulate your natural sleep system for rapid relief of insomnia.

Chapter 9: There is one factor present almost universally in people with insomnia. Their brains have become programmed to sleep poorly. Chapter 9 will teach you how this happens and why this may be the best news you hear all day. It will also teach you the second rapid insomnia relief strategy.

Chapter 10: When it comes to insomnia your mind can be a blessing or a curse. This chapter reveals how you are causing your own insomnia through unrealistic expectations and beliefs about sleep. It also teaches how your busy, thinking, worrying mind fuels the fires of insomnia and how you can put those fires out.

Chapter 11: Insomnia can be controlled. Sleep can't. Chapter 11 will give you a better understanding of sleep's slippery side and a strategy for luring sleep to bed when you feel like it's turned its back on you.

Chapter 12: Insomnia happens at night but it's a 24 hour problem. This chapter will challenge you to broaden your perspective and start looking for causes (and solutions) to your insomnia in unexpected times (and places).

Chapter 13: Stress and sleep don't get along. The problem is we're all stressed much of the time, even if it is good stress. This chapter teaches you about different types of stress and how they steal your sleep. More importantly, this chapter ends with two powerful ways to begin to undermine the impact of stress on your sleep.

Chapter 14: There is a way out of insomnia and you are in control. Chapter 14 summarizes the strategies from the 10 Laws into one place so you can begin to apply them in a systematic way. Applying these strategies can be challenging so there's also an exercise for creating a compelling vision of your best life without insomnia that you can use to motivate you as you make this vision a reality.

Chapter 15: Some sleep puzzles are just plain confusing and overwhelming. This chapter describes how we approach the Guided Sleep Discovery process in The Insomnia Clinic. It also outlines how an insomnia specialist can collaborate with you to solve your sleep puzzle using advanced sleep discovery technology.

Chapter 16: We all need a little help sometimes. The Insomnia Clinic provides the consultation and support of an insomnia expert. Chapter 16 describes the sources of sleep transformation and how they are used to bring about radical sleep transformation for clients of The Insomnia Clinic.

Chapter 17: I finally talk directly about sleep medications and how many people who start using them end up dependent. In this chapter I'll also talk about how and why you can almost certainly get free of them and hold on to satisfying sleep.

Chapter 18: What can you do to give yourself the best chance for a good night's sleep? Chapter 18 ends the book with a run down on healthy sleep habits. You'll learn how to approach things like caffeine, exercise, tobacco, food, and alcohol to set yourself up for the best sleep possible.

Your best life is waiting.

This book is about how to restore healthy natural sleep. Although it feels good to sleep, the real reason we do it is because sleep makes everything else better. WAY BETTER! When we sleep we are smarter, stronger, healthier, nicer, happier and just plain awesome. Read this book. Learn about sleep. Follow the laws of insomnia that seem right to you. Take control of your insomnia and get back to building your best life!

Wishing you blissful sleep and vibrant days!

Robert N. Glidewell
Founder, The Insomnia Clinic
Member, Sleep Health Revolution

CHAPTER 2

MY STORY PART I: INSOMNIAC TO INSOMNIA EXPERT

I'm an overachiever, a perfectionist. I like to do things well and I like things done well. I have a hard time accepting less than awesome. When my life is at its best I'm looking to learn how to make it even better. In fact, one of the most useful sayings I've come across and one that I use almost daily is, "If something is worth doing, it's worth doing wrong." Yes you read that correctly. I know the traditional version says that it's worth doing right, but that one doesn't work for me. If I do something "right" it will never get done and I'll find myself forever spinning my wheels trying to make it perfect. In fact, if you notice some typos or the grammar isn't just right in the rest of the book, it's because I decided to "do it wrong." Otherwise you wouldn't get to read it for another 10 years.

This applies to my work, my life, and my health. I want things to be the best they can be. Like all of us, I'm not always successful and there are always areas of my life I want to be different. But I'm always working to create the absolute best life possible for my family, myself, and everyone I come in contact with. I want to do this by taking as much action as possible. I don't just want things to be awesome or think about them being awesome. I want to make them awesome. That's just who I am. I'm also an insomniac.

Insomniac and Night Owl

If you ask my mother, she'll tell you about the endless nights spent awake with her baby boy who never wanted to sleep. I don't remember this so I don't think it bothered me nearly as much as it bothered her. As I grew older, my refusal to sleep turned into an inability to sleep. I was a night owl. I just wasn't sleepy when bedtime came around and couldn't fall asleep no matter how hard I tried (This is when I fell in love with the original Star Trek reruns). Other nights, I would wake up in the middle of the night and lie in bed thinking, worrying, or just wide awake for no reason. Moving to another room to sleep on the couch worked for a while. I learned to worry about my sleep in the evenings and count the hours of sleep I was losing as the night wore on. I learned of the frustration and loneliness of lying awake when everyone else was sleeping. I learned how hard it is to be the person you want to be when lack of sleep makes you so terribly tired, unmotivated, and uninterested in family, friends, work, and fun. You can imagine how well the combination of perfectionist and insomniac go together.

Perfectionist and Insomniac

I graduated high school and "celebrated" my 18th birthday in basic training for the United States Air Force. As you can guess, I fell in love, got married, and we had a beautiful baby girl the day after my 22nd birthday. I enjoyed my time in the Air Force but after almost seven years I decided to leave the Air Force and pursue my training in psychology. I completed a bachelor's degree and went straight into graduate school and began to follow the path to become a psychologist. Insomnia was a constant companion.

I wanted my life to be awesome. I wanted to be an awesome father, husband, soldier, student, etc... I did my best to push through and pretend everything was fine. But, like I said, it's hard to be the person you want to be when lack of sleep makes you so terribly tired, unmotivated, and uninterested. I was unhappy, even miserable. I was not happy with myself (nowhere near living up to my perfect expectations). I was not happy with my family or my work because I was so tired and moody.

I didn't want to think about sleep. I just wanted to focus on living my best life, but it wasn't that easy. It was impossible to live the life I wanted to live without worrying about sleep. So, over the years I tried everything I could find. Relaxation tapes, counseling, sleeping pills, alcohol, different bedtime routines, and avoiding caffeine. I'm also an anxious kind of guy (goes along with the perfectionist type) so I even tried medications for that. Nothing worked all that well.

What I realize now is that all my efforts, and the efforts of my doctors and counselors to restore healthy sleep were lacking a fundamental understanding of natural sleep and how it goes awry. What's also clear is that I did the best I could with the knowledge and tools I had available. For that matter, my healthcare providers also did their best. All their recommendations and prescriptions were appropriate and represented the standard of care at the time. However, none of this led me out of insomnia.

Discovery: Personal Sleep Transformation

Then I made a discovery that has shaped my life ever since. In the spring of 2003 I was in the middle of my doctoral training. A class on abnormal psychology and another research paper. The assignment? Pick a category of mental disorders, write a paper on it and make a presentation to the class. When I saw sleep disorders on the list I jumped at the chance to learn more. There was no other aspect of "abnormal psychology" more relevant to me personally. Here is a quote from one of the papers I ultimately wrote on sleep and insomnia:[1-2]

Regarding the treatment of sleep disturbances there is a consensus among sleep professionals that pharmacological treatments are appropriate on a short term basis to resolve acute disruptions of sleep (Morin et al., 1999). It is recognized that long term pharmacological treatment of chronic sleep disturbances is not indicated due to (a) risk of drug dependence and (b) absence of long term efficacy (i.e. sleep disturbance returns on discontinuation of the drug). For chronic sleep disturbances, behavioral treatment is recognized as having short and long-term efficacy (Morin et al., 1999). Specific behavioral treatments

19

include sleep restriction, stimulus control, sleep hygiene education, re-laxation training, positive routines, extinction/graduated extinction, and cognitive-behavior therapy.

A review paper by the American Academy of Sleep Medicine reports extant evidence on the statistical and clinical significance and durabil-ity of improvements from behavioral treatments (Morin et al., 1999). Two meta-analysis of the treatment efficacy of behavioral treatments report effect sizes ranging from .42 to .94 on several sleep variables including Sleep Onset Latency, Wake After Sleep Onset, Number of Awakenings, Total Sleep Time, and Sleep Quality. Numerous studies in this review indicate between 39 and 76 percent of subjects receiving behavioral treatment experienced clinically significant improvement depending on the criterion used to make this judgment. In terms of du-rability of treatment effects, behavioral treatments demonstrate main-tained or even improved efficacy at 3 month, 6 month, and 1 year fol-low-ups.

In the same review, Morin et al. (1999) report studies comparing the efficacy of pharmacological and behavioral treatments. Studies re-viewed indicate that behavioral and pharmacological treatments "pro-duced equivalent improvements at post treatment (mean sleep latency of 36 min), but the trajectory of change over time was different" (p. 9). In this study, pharmacological treatment produced improvements in the first week, whereas behavioral treatments showed results at the one-month follow-up. Additionally, treatment gains obtained with pharmacological treatment are not maintained at long term follow-up. Also reported are findings that when pharmacological and behavioral treatments are combined subjects "do not retain their clinical gains at follow-up as well as those treated with behavior therapy alone" (p. 10).

The evidence provided by Morin et al. (1999) provides a strong case for the efficacy of behavioral treatments for sleep disturbance; behavioral treatments produce statistically and clinically significant changes on several sleep variables and those changes are maintained over time. Based on this review the American Academy of Sleep Medicine have published practice parameters and rated each treatment according to the American Psychological Association's criteria for empirically based treatments (Chesson et al., 1999). This brings us to the second obstacle of knowledge of and training in these behavioral treatments as well as assessment and diagnosis. Several books and articles already exist to fill this need (Bootzin, Engle-Friedman, and Hazlewood, 1983; Pallesen, Nordhus, Havik, and Nielsen, 2001; Mindell, 1993; Morin, 1993; Woolfolk and McNulty, 1983).

Although the papers I wrote were clinical and "scientificy," my experiences around what I learned were deeply personal. I took what I learned about cognitive-behavioral treatments for insomnia (what I now call sleep transformation training) and began to follow them intensely in full perfectionist mode. I changed my sleep schedules. I changed the way I responded when I couldn't sleep. I began to understand my circadian rhythm and how to manipulate my internal clock. This mysterious problem called insomnia now made sense. What's more amazing, I began to experience a powerful sense of confidence and control around my sleep.

As I write this, it's been more than 10 years since I stumbled on this insomnia cure and experienced my own sleep transformation. Much of what I learned and used to overcome my own insomnia is in this book. I still struggle from time to time (believe it or not, some insomnia is normal), but my sleep and my life have been better ever since. In addition to my personal transformation, I had found my calling. I decided to become an insomnia expert.

Insomniac to Expert and Evangelist

I wasn't satisfied with my own radical sleep transformation. Why had I gone through the first 30 years of my life spinning my wheels, wrestling with insomnia, and trying to pretend like everything was okay when there was a solution hiding in the cold dark basement of science since the 1970's? For that matter, why was it hidden? Why weren't doctors and nurses and therapists shouting it from the rooftops?

The answer, as I saw it at the time, was that there was no good answer. I was a young, ambitious and zealous grad student who had just reclaimed his vigor from the jaws of insomnia. I had found my mission and I was off to save the world from insomnia and our broken healthcare system's failure to make the cure available.

From that point forward my training was focused on two goals:

- Becoming a psychologist and behavioral sleep specialist

- Getting healthcare providers to share these methods of treating insomnia without pills

I did everything I could to learn about insomnia. What causes it? What makes it better? How does it interact with health and illness? I did everything I could to learn about sleeping pills. How do they work? How are they used by insomniacs? How are they viewed and experienced by insomniacs? I also did everything I could to learn how doctors think about and interact with insomnia and sleep medication. I wanted to understand these things as deeply as possible.

I looked at thousands of scientific studies. I attended training after training and conference after conference. I wrote a dissertation on how to screen for sleep disorders in primary care[3]; I gave presentations to anyone who would listen. I continued this after graduation and after becoming licensed as a psychologist. I started my own original research and published in sleep medicine, family medicine, and neurology journals.[4-8] I started treating hundreds of insomniacs per year.

When I started this process I was optimistic and ambitious. On the heels of my personal sleep transformation, I was energized to become a world-class expert in the field of insomnia and sleep disorders. I've now done that, and it continues to be immensely gratifying to lead others through their own Guided Sleep Discovery and Radical Sleep Transformation.

I'm now energized to help even more people discover their own transformation with the launch of The Insomnia Clinic, early in 2015. You can learn more about the clinic and our exclusive systems in Chapters 15 and 16.

Unfortunately, progress toward the second goal, the one about getting healthcare providers to share these methods of treating insomnia without pills, led straight to frustration and disillusionment.

CHAPTER 3

MY STORY PART II: BIRTH OF THE SLEEP HEALTH REVOLUTION™

My frustration grew as I talked to more and more medical providers and came face to face with the realities of medical practice, the pharmaceutical industry, and our mammoth healthcare system. As I listened to the stories of more and more insomniacs I became more and more disillusioned. Too many times I had patients ask me, "Why was I never told about sleep transformation?" Too many times I heard the lament, "I only wish I'd known how to do this years ago."

The research that sleep transformation works is overwhelming but when I shared it with healthcare providers I was confronted with disbelief. They truly could not see how retraining the sleep system was possible without medication. Even if they believed in the sleep transformation program, many providers were honest about just being too busy to actively address insomnia, which they saw as a low priority. Some were even more honest and expressed their own feelings of frustration and ineffectiveness around insomnia. For other providers, resistance to sleep transformation was more a matter of mistrust or beliefs about healthcare economics. Needless to say, I was surprised to encounter this long list of obstacles to something I originally saw as so simple.

Seeing some of these complexities I entered problem solving mode. In order to join with providers and help them to overcome these real obstacles I designed the SHARP™ program, Sleep for Health, Healing, and Relapse Prevention™. SHARP is a specialized program of Radical Sleep Transformation specifically designed to assist healthcare providers in offering sleep transformation to their patients while removing as many obstacles to patient access as possible. Then I hit another barrier. As I talked to medical directors about beginning to share the SHARP program I was shocked when confronted with statements like, "Well, we can't support or endorse any program with private interests."

What!?

You can prescribe more than a billion dollars per year in sleep medications to feed the profits of massive pharmaceutical companies, but you're conflicted about offering your patients a free training program?

What!? Now *I* was in disbelief.

Respect and Understanding

As I was able to get some perspective, I began to ask why. Why were these incredibly smart and compassionate healers so uncomfortable with the non-medication option? Why was it so hard for them to believe the evidence, even when the obstacles of time, money and effectiveness were overcome? Why was a medical director threatened by integrating a formal sleep transformation training program alongside the traditional medication options?

For a while I was stumped. The men and women I was talking to were intelligent. Extremely so. They were critically thinking, compassionate individuals who have dedicated their life to serving and healing. Some of them were friends and colleagues whom I have tremendous respect for. So I went back to read those papers I wrote in grad school and I reread many of the research articles I had used to write those papers. The answers had been there all along.

- In asking medical providers to focus more on insomnia and to offer non-medication treatments I was bumping up against a major gap in medical training. Most providers have received little to no training in sleep and sleep disorders.[1-2] The best medical schools offer only few hours of training in sleep and sleep disorders while most schools include no formal training in these areas. I was also up against years of training that leads providers to give medication a preferred status over non-medication alternatives, even when medication may not be the safest or most effective option.

- I came to understand that this bias is about more than training; it is also driven by the powerful influence of pharmaceutical companies. Seth Godin, one of the most innovative thinkers in marketing, gives us some insight into the reason for this influence, "In 2003 pharmaceutical companies spent more on marketing and sales than they did on research and development. When it comes time to invest, it's pretty clear that spreading the ideas behind the medicine is more important than inventing the medicine itself."[3] Providers diligently strive to remain objective in their medical decision making. However, in 2012 they were faced with the $27 Billion influence of pharmaceutical companies.[4-5] This combination of training and influence has led providers to hold a dual standard for scientific evidence they require to support medication versus non-medication health solutions.

- We have a lot of trust and respect for the knowledge, opinions and recommendations of our healthcare providers. Providers take the power and responsibility associated with our trust in them very seriously. In order to recommend a healthcare solution they have to believe in it and trust that it is the best thing for you, their patient. It is easy for them to recommend medications because they know them; they are highly trained to evaluate and judge them. When it comes to non-medication options, most providers have almost no training, making it difficult for providers to recommend them wisely and effectively.

- Even when a provider is knowledgeable and confident about non-medication alternatives they still must navigate the challenge of limited time and competing priorities. This was hard for me to swallow at first. We're talking about people's health here, people's lives. The more I learned the more I understood the tremendous pressures providers are under, and the dysfunctional realities of the system they are required to work within. Providers would love to spend more time with you and you would probably be much happier if you didn't feel that your provider was distracted and rushed when he or she was with you. Unfortunately, our healthcare system prioritizes a brief consultative model, so until we revolt, we will be rushed and frustrated. Now, what about priorities?

- The average visit with a patient is only a few minutes long and most individuals don't go into the visit to talk about sleep. Sleep typically only comes up as related to another problem. Let's say you're in the office because of pain in your feet related to diabetes and then you also mention you're having trouble sleeping. Talk about priorities. If you have only a few minutes would you rather talk about diabetes, a problem that could kill you, rob you of your sight, or lead you to lose a foot? Or would you rather talk about your insomnia? The decision is pretty clear for most of us. Yes, sleep is important but most providers are appropriately prioritizing it in the face of more serious and urgent medical concerns.

- As if the demands of time and competing priorities weren't enough, when providers do engage insomnia they often feel ineffective. The drugs they have available have significant risks that make providers uncomfortable prescribing them in many cases. On top of their safety concerns, many providers say sleep medications just don't work that well. They say that their patients often come back dissatisfied and still struggling to sleep. Despite this, providers typically feel they don't have anything else to offer their patients. Talk about a recipe for frustration.

- I used to get excited when I heard this. "Oooh. They're unhappy with sleep medications. They want something better. I have just the thing!" I'd say to myself. My excitement was met with another obstacle. Mistrust. Providers are more and more required to act as the gatekeepers of healthcare. They must decide what is appropriate or necessary and what is not in order to act as good stewards of healthcare resources generally and their patient's financial resources specifically. This is a daunting task when you think about all the pharmaceutical, medical equipment, diagnostic, laboratory, and specialty medical service companies vying for provider attention and recommendation. They are already short on time for patients. Where are they going to find time to learn everything they need to know about the priority treatments and procedures, let alone a new non-medication solution for a frustrating but low priority health problem? Often it is easiest to defer it to outside judgment. "Is it covered by insurance?" providers would ask. They seemed to feel that if a service or product was covered by an insurance company then it was legitimate.

I've come away from these experiences with a profound respect for our healthcare providers and their service to us. They are committed, passionate, and compassionate healers who have taken on the tremendous responsibility of making high stakes decisions based on intensely complex information within the demanding requirements of a broken system. They deserve our respect, our courtesy, and our gratitude.

Unfortunately this new respect for healthcare providers has not lessened my frustration or disillusionment. Sleep is too important to be ignored or lost to higher priorities, even if they are legitimate. It is too important to be lost to convenience, disbelief, or mistrust. The burdens of undertreated insomnia in terms of finances and suffering are too great to go unchallenged.

We are in need of a Sleep Health Revolution and we must be the ones to start it.

Birth of the Sleep Health Revolution

This personal journey out of insomnia and into the complex and frustrating trenches of healthcare has shaped my belief in the necessity of a sleep health revolution. We cannot rely on drug companies whose essential goal is to sell more medication. We cannot rely on insurance companies whose primary focus is delivering the cheapest possible care. We cannot rely on our healthcare providers who are in a daily battle to provide the best care possible in the midst of a merciless system driving them away from time with patients and toward assembly line medicine.

What does a sleep health revolution look like? I'm glad you asked.

It begins by making the principles and teachings of Radical Sleep Transformation AVAILABLE to EVERYONE for FREE. This is why I've chosen to make the digital "Revolution Edition" of this book available for free. It is also why I created the SHARP program, which provides free basic sleep transformation training. These resources can be accessed here at no cost:

Laws of Insomnia "Revolution Edition":
www.coloradoinsomniaclinic.com/revolutionedition

SHARP Sleep Training Video:
www.coloradoinsomniaclinic.com/sharpsleeptraining

I've made these resources available. Now it's time for you to use them and share them using the three steps of the Sleep Health Revolution I've outlined below.

STEP 1: Take Charge of Your Own Sleep Health

Learn for yourself that sleep transformation is possible by making your own sleep health a priority. This starts with reading the rest of this book, following the recommendations to the best of your ability, and connecting with resources through The Insomnia Clinic. It may also mean starting the conversation about sleep with your healthcare provider and possibly seeing a sleep specialist. It will definitely mean investing time and possibly money in achieving maximum sleep health in support of your best life.

STEP 2: Encourage and Recruit Others to Take Charge of Their Own Sleep Health

Tell the people you know and care about that sleep transformation is possible. Help them get a free digital version of this book, show them how to access free SHARP trainings, and connect them up with The Insomnia Clinic. Thirty percent of the entire adult population complains of poor sleep. That's one in every three or about 100 million people who are kept from living their best life as a result of poor sleep. Those are 100 million people whose lives could improve if they knew how to transform their sleep. Few of these individuals have ever been offered anything other than a medication to help them sleep. Many have never spoken to their healthcare provider about poor sleep because they believe the only thing their provider has to offer them is a pill.

STEP 3: Encourage and Recruit Your Healthcare Provider to Join the Revolution

Speak with your healthcare provider. Let them know that sleep transformation is possible. Show them how their patients can get a free digital version of this book and access the free SHARP trainings. Show them how their patients can connect with The Insomnia Clinic.

Your healthcare providers respect your experience and your endorsement. Your personal experience of sleep transformation may be the most powerful way to help them overcome the many obstacles to integrating sleep transformation into their practice and offering it to their patients. If you wish they would have recommended sleep transformation to you years ago then let them know that. Imagine the number of lives you could impact if even a single one of your healthcare providers began offering sleep transformation to their patients.

Personal Invitation to the Revolution

As I write this I realize how ridiculous these goals might seem. There are many whose sleep is important enough for them to take charge of their own sleep health and many who will be so excited about their success to be willing to share with friends and family and invite them to the sleep revolution. But who is going to care enough about their own sleep health, let alone the sleep health of other individuals and their community, to spread the idea that sleep is important and we can take charge of our sleep without pills? Who is willing to begin to talk to their doctors about how they wish they had been told about the principles of sleep transformation before giving them a pill? Who is willing to encourage their doctors to join the revolution and begin sharing sleep transformation with all of their patients?

I'm hoping that you are. I'm hoping you're willing to join me and many others in the revolution. In fact, whether you or not you think of yourself as a revolutionary, you joined when you started reading this book. The information in this book can take you a long way toward personal sleep transformation, maybe all the way. However, the path of sleep transformation can be challenging to walk alone, which is why I created The Insomnia Clinic.

The Insomnia Clinic

I know there is a solution to every sleep problem. I know this because I found my own sleep solution and since that time I've helped hundreds of others find their solution. But the number of people I can help on my own is limited. This reality led me to build The Insomnia Clinic, which is focused on helping thousands of people a year through my systems of Guided Sleep Discovery and Radical Sleep Transformation.

You can learn more about the clinic and these systems in Chapters 15 and 16. For now I'll tell you that The Insomnia Clinic brings you sleep wellness coaches and licensed healthcare providers trained as insomnia specialists who can walk you through your own Guided Sleep Discovery and Radical Sleep Transformation using revolutionary educational and clinical programs. While I created The Insomnia Clinic to help you understand your sleep problem and find your sleep solution, you are only one of an estimated 100 million Americans who struggle with insomnia, many if not most of whom would love to know about sleep transformation. I like to think of The Insomnia Clinic as a training camp for revolutionaries. My goal is to help you sleep better so you can start living your best life. When you sleep well you...

- Think more clearly

- Have more positive moods

- Enjoy work and family more

- Have more energy and motivation

- Become more active and engaged in the things you value

My hope is that this experience will inspire you to tell others and encourage them to take charge of their own sleep health. Also, that you will be inspired to talk to your doctors and begin to break down the biases that have prevented people like you with insomnia from knowing that sleep transformation was possible much sooner.

PART 1

UNDERSTANDING INSOMNIA AND SOLVING
THE PUZZLE OF POOR SLEEP

CHAPTER 4

LAW #1: SLEEP IS CRITICALLY ESSENTIAL

How many news headlines, social media posts, or internet ads have you seen about sleep or insomnia over the last month? It seems everywhere you turn there are stories of the effects of insomnia, sleep deprivation, or other sleep disorders. What's the basic message of these stories? Insomnia changes lives and it changes every area of life. There are so many of these stories and they are so popular for two reasons. First, you're not alone. One of every three adults in the United States complains of insomnia. Second, sleep is critically essential for every function of the brain and body. This means that inadequate or disrupted sleep compromises the most basic workings of your brain and body in a way that fundamentally undermines your ability to live your best life.

Changes in the brain and body that result from poor sleep are almost always in the direction of restricting or limiting health, performance, relationships, and overall happiness. Over time, those who struggle with insomnia find their lives seeming to shrink around them, becoming less than they had imagined. If you have struggled with insomnia for any length of time you may be more familiar with the effects of insomnia than you would like. Depending on the shape of your insomnia, you may be seeing more or less of these effects.

"It's very controlling....like if I want to have company....I could have
a bad night...then I won't feel like having them over."

-Vicky, Age 29, Insomnia Interview[1]

Maybe you've noticed you're not spending time with friends or doing things you used to enjoy because you just don't have the energy (or interest) anymore. Maybe you've stopped making commitments out of fear that you won't be able to keep them if you've had a bad night. Maybe you're feeling isolated or misunderstood because no one seems to understand how you could have such a big problem with something as natural as sleep. Maybe you've started sleeping in a separate bed to keep from disturbing your partner during the night.

Insomnia has a way of distancing us from our most important and valued connections. Sometimes this happens because of a lack of energy and motivation to do the simple things that keep us connected like picking up the phone or saying yes to the unexpected invitation for coffee or lunch. Insomnia is still misunderstood with many still doubting if it is real or believing it's a sign of mental illness. When you don't "look" sick on the outside it's hard for others to understand the burden of insomnia. Because of this, too often I hear stories of people who are embarrassed to talk with their family, friends, and even their healthcare providers about their insomnia.

"How a Bad Night's Sleep
Can Derail Your Career"

– The Fiscal Times[2]

Maybe you are not as sharp at work as you used to be, finding yourself struggling with decisions and less creative than you used to be. Maybe things that used to come easy are harder to do and take longer to get done. Maybe the excitement you used to have about work has turned to boredom, or worse, loathing. Maybe you're too tired to be in front on the fast track and now find yourself just trying to keep up.

There is a word for this – presenteeism - and insomnia can be a major cause. It means you go to work but aren't really "showing up." Insomnia causes an average of almost 30 days and thousands of dollars in lost productivity per person each year.[3-4] At the end of the day, insomnia equals less satisfaction at work while getting paid less and receiving fewer promotions.[5]

"Sleepy Wife May Take it Out on Hubby"

– NBC News on TODAY.com[6]

Maybe you're moody and irritable and just not as nice to the people you care about as you (and they) wish you could be. Maybe you're too tired to rise to that invitation from your kiddos for another game of Twister. Maybe you're having trouble putting your finger on it but just know you are not the person you want to be.

Relationships and parenting are challenging even when we are at our best. Insomnia drains our energy and brings down our mood, making the normally joyful demands of being a partner and parent seem like a chore. Under the burden of insomnia it's also easy to be less appreciative of the good things and people around us. Over time our relationships can come to seem like something we must push through, leaving us feeling like we are surviving rather than thriving when around the people we love.

"Could Insomnia Pose a Cancer Risk?"

– The OZ BLOG on www.DOCTOROZ.com[7]

Maybe your sleep problem is taking a toll on your health, causing or putting you at risk for illness. Or, maybe you've been injured or are already struggling to reclaim your health from some type of illness. Maybe you're worried that your sleep problem is keeping you from healing.

Of the top 10 health concerns, men and women have six of them in common. They are Heart Disease, Cancer, Stroke, Diabetes/Obesity, Osteoporosis, and Depression. Every one of these is connected to insomnia and sleep deprivation in some way. It's easy to become overwhelmed with worry over health concerns. But worrying doesn't really take you very far. Instead, focus on what you can do to empower yourself and take control where you can. As you read on, you will learn that insomnia is absolutely an area where you can be empowered to take control.

Sometimes it is difficult for family, friends, and coworkers to understand what is so difficult about sleeping and how insomnia can change lives. It's important to know that the effect of your insomnia on your life depends on several things. Some of these things are:

- **Your personal sensitivity.** Some people are just more sensitive to the effects of insomnia than others.

- **How often you have insomnia.** Trouble sleeping once a week may be a nuisance, trouble sleeping five nights a week may be affecting your relationships, work, and social life.

- **The intensity of your insomnia.** Are you losing hours of sleep a night? Are you getting plenty of sleep but just feel like its light and restless? The amount of sleep you're losing and the quality of your sleep can have a powerful influence on how you feel and function during the day.

- **The cause or causes of your insomnia.** Body clock problems, breathing problems, restless legs, and stress, are just a few of the causes of insomnia. The cause of your insomnia strongly influences what kind of insomnia you have and how it affects you.

In this book I will share a few stories of how insomnia takes a toll on life and health but first I would like you to take a minute and use the space over the next couple of pages to create *Your Sleep Story*.

1. How long have you had insomnia? Do you have any thoughts about *why* you have it?

   _____

   _____

2. What do other people say or think about your insomnia? Are you comfortable talking to friends, family, or healthcare providers about your insomnia?

   _____

   _____

3. What is it like for you when you try to go to sleep at night or when you wake up during the night? What are the thoughts, feelings, and body sensations that arise when you have trouble sleeping?

   _____

   _____

4. How does your insomnia affect your life during the day?

   _____

   _____

   a. Is your work or school performance and enjoyment what you want and need it to be?

      _____

      _____

   b. Are you the person you want to be in relationships with friends and family? With your children?

      _____

      _____

c. Do you have the energy and passion to do the things you love? Or are you just surviving?

_____

_____

Take a moment now to look over your sleep story. What are your thoughts? Are the effects of insomnia in your life more or less than you might have imagined before writing it? You may be surprised that you are doing as well as you are. On the other hand, maybe you're thinking you should be doing better than you are, despite your insomnia. Whatever your sleep story, I want you to know that insomnia is a real problem that has real consequences for health, happiness, success, and relationships.

With that said, I also want you to know that insomnia is a problem that can be understood and effectively treated in almost every situation. Yes, insomnia can take a heavy toll on your health and relationships. Yes, insomnia can drain you of the energy, motivation, and joy necessary to keep you vital and vibrant in your work, family, and social life. Yes, 90% of people get significantly better in a matter of weeks once they make the decision to take control of their insomnia. Yes, 40% of people will be able to completely eliminate their insomnia, many without sleeping pills.

I hope you've found this book early in the process of insomnia affecting your life. But, wherever you are, know that you can take control of insomnia. You can reclaim healthy natural sleep. You can reclaim your life, your happiness, and your health. Now it's time to take a look at the pieces of your insomnia puzzle.

CHAPTER 5

LAW #2: INSOMNIA HAS MANY CAUSES

Sleep is an indicator of wellness. Sleeping well or poorly can be a general reflection of your overall wellness, health, and life satisfaction. This is good and bad. Good because when you have a sleep problem it can be an early sign that something is getting out of balance in your health or in your life. Bad because it means there are so many things that can cause insomnia.

Basically, anything that makes you mentally, physically, or emotionally uncomfortable has the potential to cause insomnia. This can lead to quite a puzzle to unravel when trying to find the causes and the right solutions. The puzzle becomes quite complicated when your insomnia has multiple causes or when your insomnia is blamed on the wrong cause.

What if there is more than one problem causing your insomnia?

It would sure be nice if problems were handed out one at a time in a neat and orderly fashion. I like it quite a bit when someone comes in with a simple insomnia that we can fix easily in just one or two visits. Sometimes I wish more people would come for help when their insomnia is just starting, before it has really begun to take a toll on their life.

Unfortunately, we humans are pretty complicated. Most of the insomnia problems I see have more than one cause. Sometimes the issue that caused insomnia to start is different from the one that keeps it going. It's not unusual to sleep somewhat better with one treatment and find that another problem is keeping sleep from getting all the way better. I find that when all the reasons for insomnia are given full attention, the chances of getting fully better increase dramatically.

What if the cause of your insomnia is not what you think it is?

I talk to people almost every week who have been trying to find the right treatment for insomnia for years, even decades, only to learn that their insomnia was really a symptom of another problem. Sleep improves once the main problem is addressed. People are grateful to be sleeping better and feeling better but frustrated that they spent so much time, energy, and money on the wrong treatments. Here are a couple of examples:

What if you have a body clock problem?

The most common reason I see for sleep medications not working is a body clock problem that is pretending to be a simple insomnia problem. In simple insomnia, a person's difficulty getting to sleep or staying asleep is due to the brain having bad programming or simply being too activated. Medications for insomnia are designed to help with this problem. When there's a body clock problem you will have trouble falling asleep or staying asleep that is caused by an entirely different part of the brain being turned on at the wrong time. If you take an insomnia medication that works on the insomnia part of the brain but you actually have a body clock problem then it makes sense why those medications either don't work or don't get you the results you're looking for.

Causes of Insomnia

Stress or Anxiety

Chronic Pain

Sleep Apnea

Asthma or Allergies

Prostate Problems

Body Clock Problems

Menopause

Depression

Medications

"Programmed" Insomnia

Many, many more...

What if you have a breathing problem while sleeping?

Everybody knows what sleep apnea looks like right? Breathing problems at night only happen in people who snore extremely loud or are extremely overweight. Wrong.[1] We have started to learn over the last many years that sleep apnea comes in many shapes and sizes. As a matter of fact, women with sleep apnea are likely to have no snoring or obvious breathing problems at all during the night. Instead they are often diagnosed with insomnia and depression for many years before anyone suspects they might have trouble breathing during the night. Nowadays, any good sleep specialist will recommend an overnight sleep study for anyone with chronic insomnia that doesn't get better with medication or sleep transformation training.

How do I solve my insomnia puzzle?

Finding the pieces of your insomnia puzzle is the first step to sleeping better. Unless you know the shape of the pieces and what part of the picture they hold, the search for the right insomnia solution is a shot in the dark. But how do you figure out those pieces? Some of you may be able to do this on your own, while others may need to follow a formal Guided Sleep Discovery process with the help of an insomnia expert. This basic sleep discovery exercise is one simple thing you can do right away:

Basic Sleep Discovery Exercise

1. Make a list of ALL the possible causes of insomnia you believe matter for you.

2. Rate how much of your insomnia (0% to 100%) is caused by each item on your list.

3. Rewrite your list in order of most important (highest %) to least important.

4. Decide what action you will take for item #1 on your list to either:

    a. Prove it is, in fact, the most important cause, OR

    b. Fix or change it in a way that will improve your sleep.

As an example, let's say you think that a busy mind is the biggest reason for trouble sleeping at the beginning and middle of the night. You've already been keeping a list by the bed to write down thoughts or worries and have not found this useful. Since that strategy has not been working you might try something else. Relaxation/meditation or a gratitude journal is both proven to change the activity of the mind when trying to sleep.

For another example, what if back pain is the most important cause of your problem? In that case, depending on the specifics of the pain, Step 4 might include any of the following options:

- 20 minutes of stretching or yoga in the evening

- Take an OTC pain medication before bed

- Contact a sleep specialist to learn how to strengthen natural sleep

- Ask your primary care provider how to best manage nighttime pain

- Ask your primary care doctor for referral to a pain specialist

Going through the process of the basic sleep discovery exercise can help you understand your insomnia in a totally different way. It can help you feel like you have more control over your insomnia. It can also help to guide you in your search for an insomnia solution that really works for you.

While many people can and do solve their insomnia puzzle on their own, sometimes the puzzle is just too complicated or confusing to solve without some expert help. In The Insomnia Clinic, when we sit down with you at your first appointment we start the conversation with an attitude of, "Let's figure this thing out together." This attitude contains four critical components for success. These are:

- **You are an expert** – You are the one who has lived your insomnia. You know yourself best. You know what has and has not worked for you. You know what you are willing and able to do to find your insomnia solution.

- **Your clinician is an expert** – Your clinician has advanced training in sleep and insomnia.

- **You are no longer alone** – Your clinician is a partner. Like a jigsaw puzzle, solving your insomnia puzzle will be faster and more enjoyable with a partner. Beginning with the very first visit, we strive to break down feelings of isolation and disconnection caused by insomnia.

- **Your insomnia puzzle can be solved** – With our combined expertise and advanced technology for understanding sleep and insomnia, there is a solution to every insomnia problem.

If you have tried more than one strategy (pills, relaxation, etc...) and are not totally satisfied with your sleep, it's probably time for you to speak with a specialist who can walk you through a Guided Sleep Discovery process. This will help you look closely at the nature of your sleep problem to identify the cause or causes.

CHAPTER 6

LAW #3: INSOMNIA HAS A LIFE OF ITS OWN

Overall, insomnia means any problem sleeping or feeling unrested even when you do sleep, no matter why it is happening. This last point - no matter why it is happening - has been the focus of a civilized argument in the healthcare community about what insomnia is and what it is not. Is it just a symptom of other problems or an independent problem? This argument is important because how you (and your healthcare provider) think about this argument will directly affect...

- What you do to fix your insomnia (if anything), and

- What treatments you and your healthcare provider consider.

When you believe Insomnia is a symptom (and why you shouldn't)

If you believe that your insomnia is just a symptom of a "primary problem" (pain, anxiety, depression, shift work, etc...) then you and your healthcare provider probably won't do anything to directly fix it. If you do choose to do something it will probably be limited to knocking you out with sleeping pills so you can get some sleep despite having the "primary problem." This may get you some sleep but it doesn't really count as fixing your sleep problem because sleeping pills truly are just a treatment for symptoms. This is problematic because I often talk to people who have basically given up on fixing their insomnia. The conversation usually goes something like this.

"You're a sleep expert?"

"Yep, I help people fix insomnia without pills."

"I wake up every night and it takes me hours to get back to sleep."

"Yeah? That must really take its toll."

"It does! I am so tired and moody all the time. I have CRS syndrome."

"CRS?"

"You know. CRS...can't remember shit."

We both laugh.

"Sounds tough. What do you do to try to sleep better?"

"Oh, I know why I don't sleep. I have _____ (insert "primary problem" here)."

They say this in a way that tells me they have given up. I used to continue the conversation by sharing some of the research that has repeatedly shown that insomnia has a life of its own and that if you treat it you will sleep better. I stopped doing this. Every time I said anything of this sort, they would get a glazed look in their eyes as they listened politely. Then they would say something like, "Yeah. Well I know my insomnia is because of _____."

Ultimately I came to understand that what they were really saying was, "There is no point in me even thinking about trying to fix my insomnia. I have no control over this thing causing me to sleep poorly so I have no control over my insomnia." Now, I don't want to minimize the importance of things like pain or depression and I am not saying that those things don't cause poor sleep.

What I am saying and what I hope you will get from this chapter is that, in my experience, "primary problems" are almost never the only cause of insomnia and targeted non-medication treatment can almost always lead to significantly better sleep. As a bonus, when you sleep better your ability to cope with and recover from the "primary problem" gets better. Keep reading. The rest of this chapter will show you the power you have to fix insomnia when you believe it has a life of its own.

When you believe insomnia has a life of its own

To show you why insomnia is not just a symptom, I'll share the story of Barbara. A friend recommended she try one of my online programs (TERRA Sleep®; www.terrasleep.com) when it was in the testing phase. Just to let you know, the program she participated in consisted of a 36 minute video training and use of Certified Pure Therapeutic Grade essential oils (think lavender). Her experience will show you how powerful even low-intensity sleep transformation programs for insomnia can be.

Barbara is a 46 year old homemaker and mother whose 10 year struggle with pain and insomnia severely limited her ability to care for her home and family. In fact, many days her pain and fatigue would keep her in bed all day. Her sleep problems continued despite use of sleeping pills.

Essential oils had helped her break free of pain medications in the past and she very much wanted to get free of sleeping medications as well. Although she did experience somewhat better sleep with essential oils she still found herself struggling to sleep and dependent on sleeping medication.

Within three weeks of starting the sleep transformation program she was sleeping 1-2 hours more each night and taking 50% less sleep medication. She was sleeping deeper and started dreaming again. She was waking up less during the night and says she might not wake up at all if only her husband would stop snoring. Her better sleep has meant less pain and she now finds that, "my bad days don't keep me down as long." Her memory is improved, she's not so hard on herself, and she is much more positive. Now getting to bed sooner and getting up earlier, she has so much more time in the day to enjoy the life she could previously only watch from the sidelines.

In only three weeks, Barbara radically improved her sleep pattern and reduced the amount of sleep medications she needed despite her pain. These changes in her sleep fundamentally transformed her life while awake. In her words, "The sleep program catapulted my ability to make changes I've been struggling with for years."

When you believe that insomnia has a life of its own, you will actively look for things that will make a difference and you will actively try new things until you find what works for you. Barbara started with essential oils because she experienced so much success with these for her pain problem. When she got only partial benefit from oils for sleep she didn't give up. Instead, when the opportunity to participate in my program came up, she jumped at the chance. Before I move on to the next chapter, I want to close with a discussion of how insomnia interacts with other health problems.

No Excuses. It really doesn't matter what's disturbing your sleep

Just to make it painfully clear that insomnia has a life of its own, here are a few tidbits from the research. Fifteen years ago, a colleague of mine named Kenneth Lichstein[1] and his associates published a study of older adults with a variety of health problems. Health problems of participants in this study included arthritis, depression, chronic respiratory disease (COPD, Asthma), neuropathy, anxiety disorders, prostate disease, and neurologic diseases (stroke, Parkinson's, epilepsy). Here's what is truly amazing about this particular study. To get into the study, the research had to determine that the participant's insomnia was caused by their other health problem. Despite their other health problems, these people reported better sleep quality and spent less time awake during the night after participating in only four sessions of sleep transformation training. Other studies of sleep transformation training for insomnia occurring with other specific health problems show the same result.

Chronic Pain

There are many types of pain (arthritis, fibromyalgia, neuropathy, back pain, cancer pain, etc...) and they can all cause poor sleep. In fact, up to 88% of people with chronic pain have significant insomnia.[2] The good news is that even when insomnia is caused by pain, sleep transformation training for insomnia helps people to fall asleep easier, spend less time awake throughout the night, and simply have better quality sleep.[3] As a side note, 30% of people with pain who participate in insomnia treatment started sleeping well enough that they chose to stop using sleep medications.[3] Additionally, in some cases, participation in insomnia treatment not only led to improved sleep but also less pain.[4]

Depression

When sleep behavior changes are added to treatment for depression, two amazing things happen. Compared to people with depression who receive depression treatment alone, depressed people who engage treatment for depression and insomnia at the same time are five times more likely to eliminate insomnia and twice as likely to eliminate depression.[5]

Sleep and Cancer

Compared to women who did not receive treatment for insomnia, when women with breast cancer that was causing or worsening insomnia participated in sleep transformation training, they reported better sleep, less need for sleep medication, less depression, less anxiety, and generally greater quality of life.[6] Women who treated their insomnia also reduced the number of nights per week they used sleep medication. Women who did not treat their insomnia ended up taking sleep medication more often.

Anxiety

When sleep behavior changes are added to treatment for anxiety disorders, the effect is similar to that described above for depression.[7] First, non-medication treatment for insomnia leads to better sleep. Second, individuals with anxiety who also treat their insomnia experience greater benefits from anxiety treatment than those individuals who did not treat their insomnia. One more thing - treatment of anxiety alone usually fails to eliminate insomnia. This means that, if you have anxiety, you will probably not get all the way better unless you also do something specifically to make your sleep better.

Sleep Apnea

This one is tricky. Breathing problems at night can cause insomnia.[8] I mean, how well can you really sleep if you're not breathing right? The problem is that most people (and their doctors) believe that fixing the breathing problem will fix the insomnia. Well, this is a specific area of interest for me. I was helping people with sleep disorders for a couple of years and kept having people with sleep apnea come to me in the clinic and say one of two things.

- I can't fall asleep with my CPAP (Continuous Positive Airway Pressure) machine on

- I'm using my CPAP every night but I still sleep poorly and feel poorly during the day

Hearing these statements enough times led me to believe that the insomnia problem was separate from the sleep apnea. It had a life of its own. So I started researching this issue. My findings were published in the journal Sleep Medicine in 2014.[9] What I and a few others have found is that many people with sleep apnea continue to sleep poorly even after their sleep apnea is treated. Additionally, when people with sleep apnea add targeted sleep transformation training for insomnia, their insomnia improves.

Alcohol Abuse and Dependence

When individuals who have used large amounts of alcohol regularly for long periods of time decide to stop drinking, it can take up to four years for their sleep patterns to return to normal.[10] This is troublesome because the presence of insomnia significantly increases the risk of relapse back into drinking. It is even more troublesome because the most common treatment for insomnia, sleep medications, are not available to them. Almost all prescription sleep medications cause dependence and are at risk of being abused. Accordingly, doctors and alcoholics avoid these kinds of medications. So, what are they to do?

Several studies have shown that use of various types of sleep transformation training for insomnia can improve the sleep of recovering alcoholics during the first couple of years after deciding to stop drinking. [10] These studies show that a few weeks of individual, group, or self-help treatment led to better sleep quality, falling asleep faster, waking up less, spending less time awake during the night, and fewer problematic thoughts and beliefs about sleep.

I'm healthy, I'm just too old

What's that saying about old dogs? They can't learn new tricks? Well, you're not a dog and that old saying is a bunch of nonsense anyway. Although we tend to sleep lighter and wake up more than when we were younger, this change in sleep as we age is not an automatic recipe for insomnia. Many older adults (if you're over 60 you're in this category) are completely happy with their sleep even though they sleep lighter and wake up more often than they used to. With that said, the frequency of insomnia does increase as we get older and this increase is mainly associated with the number of health problems we have and the number of medications we take. This doesn't mean you have to sit back and take it.

Remember that study I mentioned earlier? Just to refresh, forty-four older adults with health problems like arthritis, depression, COPD, Asthma, neuropathy, anxiety disorders, prostate disease, stroke, Parkinson's, and epilepsy reported better sleep quality and spent less time awake during the night after participating in only four sessions of sleep transformation training.[1] That same year, another group of researchers found almost the same thing.[11] Another group of older adults with insomnia and a variety of other health problems participated in their version of sleep transformation training, and guess what happened? When these adults participated in an eight week class, 73% of them had a major transformation in their sleep. When another group instead watched a video of the classes at home, 50% had major sleep transformation. What did this transformation look like? They fell asleep faster, spent less time awake during the night, had better quality sleep, and built up healthier beliefs about sleep. They also said they had better moods, were more social, felt more energetic and had more vitality during the day.

I've had trouble sleeping my whole life/decades

Many individuals who have insomnia for a long time fall into beliefs that if a problem has been around for a long time, then it will take a long time to fix and may not be able to be fixed at all. That may be true for some problems but not for insomnia. My experience in The Insomnia Clinic is that even the most long lasting insomnia problem can often be transformed in a matter of weeks. I also heard a colleague speak about his research on an online sleep transformation program at a conference recently. He has information on more than 1000 individuals with insomnia who have participated in the program and he found something very interesting. The chances of getting better using his online sleep transformation program were the same no matter how long the insomnia had been around and no matter how severe the insomnia.[12]

How can this be?

This goes back to the title of this chapter: Insomnia has a life of its own. Because this is true, because insomnia is at least partially if not largely separate from your other health problems, there are specific things that you can do to transform it. The next section focuses on the three strategies most likely to bring you rapid insomnia relief.

- How to approach or respond to your insomnia

- How to strengthen your natural sleep system

- How to reverse negative insomnia programming

Keep reading. You're on the road to your own personal sleep transformation. For now, I encourage you to see your insomnia as something separate and in addition to other health problems. Having this view will support thinking and action patterns most likely to get you sleeping better faster. You can choose to fix your sleep and your sleep will get better...even if you have other problems. If you can change the way you see your sleep problem, you're only one step away from seeing the power you have to get better.

PART 2

RADICAL SLEEP TRANSFORMATION™:
RAPID INSOMNIA RELIEF

CHAPTER 7

LAW #4: INSOMNIA IS A TRICKY PROBLEM (FIVE OBSTACLES TO SUCCESS)

Starting in chapter 8, I will finally start teaching you the two most powerful ways to transform insomnia. But first I want to inoculate you against the five attitudes, approaches, and misunderstandings most likely to be obstacles to your success. Insomnia is a tricky problem in so many ways. There are many natural and intuitive ways to respond when you have trouble sleeping. Unfortunately the responses that seem to make the most sense usually worsen insomnia rather than make it better. On top of that, it's easy to do those things that make insomnia worse while the things most likely to get you sleeping better can be quite challenging and seem to make no sense on the surface. This chapter takes a close look at the tricky ways of insomnia.

If it makes sense, it's probably the wrong thing to do.

When you have trouble sleeping you probably don't just sit back and whine about it. You probably do things to try to fix it or at least compensate for the effects. You do things that make sense like:

- Trying to make up for the sleep you know you'll lose, you start spending more time in bed by going to bed earlier or trying to sleep in later

- You start napping to make up for lost sleep

- More tired than usual in the evenings, you may have started dozing in front of the TV

- Knowing it will be a struggle, you stay up later than usual because you now dread going to bed

- Fatigued because of poor sleep (or little sleep) you become less active, you turn down those invitations from friends for weekend mountain biking and stop going to the gym

- Trying harder and harder to get the sleep you desperately want and need

- You try to distract yourself from sleeplessness or at least make it less miserable by doing things like watching TV or movies or listening to audiobooks or podcasts in bed

When these things don't work, a sense of powerlessness over sleep begins to creep in. Thinking, planning, and worrying about sleep and the consequences of sleep loss make it ever harder to sleep. Here are a few ways that thoughts and emotions cause even more trouble sleeping:

- You start worrying about sleep in the evenings and may dread going to bed

- Unable to sleep, worries about how poorly you'll feel tomorrow start to play in your mind

- Worry about health consequences

- Unpleasantness of these thoughts slowly takes you farther from sleep the longer they continue

All these things make sense and they are the universal responses to trouble sleeping. In fact, if you are doing one or more of these you could even consider yourself normal. The problem is that they actually don't work.

Although they might help you feel somewhat better, they will almost certainly make your sleep problem worse and keep the insomnia going month after month after month.

The "Right" Things Make No Sense

You've probably read or heard some of the basic recommendations about how to fix insomnia.

"Get out of bed if you can't sleep within 15-20 minutes"

"Get up at the same time every day...even on the weekends"

These are good recommendations. If you follow them they will probably help you sleep better. When I ask people to follow recommendations like these I often get what I call the crazy face. This is a face with the eyes wide and lips pursed in a doubtful way that says, "You're crazy. How do I get out of here?" They don't say this of course, at least not until they are sleeping better and they know me and feel comfortable sharing with me their first impression. Instead they say something like:

"If I get out of bed I'll just wake up more. Then I'll never get to sleep."

"At least I'm resting when I'm in bed. If I get out of bed I'll feel even worse the next day."

"Why would I get up early on the weekends? That's when I get my best sleep!"

Most of the things that people can use to transform their sleep patterns without pills are like this. They are powerful and there is a mountain of research to show they work but they seem like exactly the opposite of what should be done. In fact, they go against our very instincts of how to respond to a sleep problem. Have you ever read an article or blog post that gives you sleep recommendations and just thought to yourself,

"That's just stupid"? Welcome to the club. You're right. They sound like nonsense! The problem is they are powerful nonsense. Stupid does not mean ineffective. If that's not bad enough, there is another thing that gets in the way of doing the right things.

It's Easy to do The "Right" Things Wrong

Any time we have to DO something we try to "make it our own" by adjusting and modifying it so it fits our unique lifestyle and needs. This just makes sense, right? Yes, unless HOW you do the thing is an essential part of whether or not you get what you want out of it. For example, negative sleep programming is an almost universal part of insomnia and the Escape, Hang Out, Try Again technique (see LAW #6: Insomnia is a Programming Problem) is the most effective way we know to "reprogram" for great sleep. But, this technique has to be done in exactly the right way for the reprogramming to occur. Basically this technique involves four steps:

1. Get out of bed if you can't sleep within 15-20 minutes.

2. Hang out in another room for 15-20 minutes.

3. Go back to bed and try again.

4. Repeat the previous steps as needed.

Sounds simple enough right? Well, talking about doing a thing is much easier than actually doing that thing. Unfortunately, there are about a hundred ways to mess it up so it doesn't actually do the job of reprogramming. Here are a few of the most common ways you could modify the "get out of bed" rule so that it doesn't work.

-   Get out of bed only to fall asleep on the couch or recliner in the other room.

-   Wait too long, until you get frustrated and uncomfortable, to get out of bed.

-   Just stay in bed and read or watch TV, rather than go to another room.

- Just sit on the edge of the bed for a minute and then lie back down.

Each of these changes to the Escape, Hang Out, and Try Again technique makes sense but they will likely undermine the success of the whole process. Let me get a little more specific about what I'm saying. The point of the Escape, Hang Out, and Try Again process is to prevent or at least minimize the amount of time you spend in bed awake or uncomfortable. Why? Because every minute you lie in bed awake is a minute your brain is learning to be awake in bed. If you spend an hour lying awake in bed thinking, planning, and worrying, then that is an hour that your brain is learning to be awake and thinking (rather than sleeping) when you're in bed.

Here's how this might play out step by step. Let's say you're lying in bed awake and after 20 minutes or so you think to yourself, "Just a little bit longer and I'll fall asleep." And then another 10 minutes goes by, and then another 10. After 40 minutes you decide to finally get up (because that's what you're supposed to do right?). That's good. You should get out of bed. However, you're not likely to get the full benefit from this strategy because every minute you stayed in bed your brain just became MORE programmed for insomnia and all you got out of the deal was 40 minutes of lying in bed without sleep.

This same unfortunate reality applies to the whole idea of staying in bed because, "at least I'm resting." Every minute you lie in bed "resting" is a minute you are training your brain that it doesn't need to sleep when you get into bed, only rest. So, by settling for rest you teach the brain that it doesn't have to go into those brain waves of restful satisfying sleep.

If you look at any list of sleep recommendations, there are probably 10 ways to do them wrong, which means misunderstand or modify them in a way that keeps them from doing the thing they were intended to do. My point? Follow the instructions for the exercises in this book to the best of your ability without changing them, and you will give yourself the best chance of blissful sleep. Even if you do the right things the right way, there are still a couple of obstacles.

Insomnia won't go away overnight...but maybe after 14 days.

Not only is it easy to mess these techniques up, you also have to do them consistently and for a long enough period of time to get the benefit. In most cases, you will have to make the right changes in the right way and stick to them for at least 14 days to begin to see the benefits. Even years-long insomnia can start to change dramatically within 14 days. However, it's often difficult to stick to these changes, which can be challenging.

Honestly, there is kind of a setup for failure here. Some of the sleep change strategies are hard to do, either because they are unpleasant or they involve having you do (at least temporarily) things that don't make sense or require you to fight your natural tendency, things like stay up past the time when you first feel sleepy or get out of bed before you feel you've have had enough sleep.

Realistically, you have to be able and willing to go through some discomfort in the beginning in order to make it through the first phase of sleep transformation training for insomnia. This is difficult if you're trying to do it on your own and you're not totally sure you are doing it right. It is also difficult if you're not sure if the discomfort you are experiencing is normal or a sign that you're making your insomnia worse.

I've Tried That and It doesn't Work For Me

One of the most unfortunate things that happens with insomnia is that people become convinced that sleep transformation training doesn't work. Or, at least it doesn't work for them. This happens for all of the reasons I just talked about. The things that will fix a sleep problem seem like exactly the wrong things to do. If you do the right things, there is a chance that you're not doing them right. If you're doing them right, it may feel like you're doing them wrong because they can cause some significant discomfort and they take a little while to start working.

I can't tell you how often I talk to people in The Insomnia Clinic who feel they've tried everything and think their sleep is hopelessly broken. Most think they have tried sleep transformation training and cognitive-behavioral therapy for insomnia, but really they have barely scratched the surface. After a short conversation, probably only 1 out of 100 has actually done the right things in the right way for long enough to have really had an impact on their insomnia.

This is good news! It means that there is hope. Chances are that you're one of the 99 who can benefit from formal sleep transformation training with the right support and instruction. It means that there may be a fairly simple way for you to quickly take control of insomnia without more medication.

CHAPTER 8

LAW #5: INSOMNIA IS A POWER PROBLEM

Sleep power is your brain's ability to fall asleep, stay asleep, and sleep deeply. While you're awake, a chemical called adenosine is building up in your brain. The more adenosine you have, the more "sleep power" you have. Falling asleep and staying asleep are part of a fairly complicated process in which a bunch of brain areas that are responsible for keeping you awake must be turned off. It takes a large amount of sleep power to turn them off. So, the more sleep power you can create, the sleepier you will be at bedtime, and the easier it will be to fall asleep, sleep deeply, stay asleep, and return to sleep. If you're serious about better sleep then you want to generate as much sleep power as possible.

Building Resistance to Disruption

Sleep power is essential for making you resistant to things that can interrupt or disrupt sleep. Remember Barbara from Chapter 6? Barbara struggled with insomnia and chronic pain. Boosting sleep power played a critical role in her overcoming insomnia despite her pain. Fortunately, her experience was not unique. Boosting sleep power can help you overcome insomnia despite a variety of health problems including bladder problems, anxiety, depression, and many other "primary" problems. Here's how I think about it. If you're a great sleeper with chronic pain, pain will disrupt your sleep a little bit. But, if you're a poor sleeper with chronic pain, the pain can destroy what little sleep you do get. You see, the stronger your natural sleep system (i.e. the more sleep power you have), the more resistant you will be to any kind of interruptions or disturbance. In the rest of this chapter I will introduce you to four "power boosts" that will strengthen your natural sleep system and make you more resistant to anything that threatens your sleep.

4 Ways to Boost Your Sleep Power

You can boost sleep power by controlling when you go to bed, controlling when you get up in the morning, controlling how much time you spend in bed, and controlling how you nap. The next several pages describe these four ways of boosting sleep power. They are also described in the SHARP sleep transformation training video (www.coloradoinsomniaclinic.com/sharpsleeptraining).

Power Boost #1: When to Go to Bed

This may seem like a trick question but...how do you decide when to go to bed? Do you go to bed because...

- You're bored

- You have to get up at a certain time

- Your bed partner goes to bed

- You're "tired"

- You can't wait for the day to end

- It's a comfortable place to hang out

If you want to have maximum sleep power and give yourself the best chance of falling asleep quickly and easily, there's only one reason to go to bed and that's when you're sleepy. You may feel like you're extremely sleepy but then go to bed and have the experience of becoming more awake or just unable to sleep. This can be caused by negative sleep programming, which you can fix with the use of specific sleep reprogramming techniques (see LAW #6: Insomnia is a Programming Problem in the next chapter). However, you may also be confusing sleepiness with being fatigued or tired.

When you're sleepy you will typically have trouble keeping your eyes open and may even start dozing off accidentally if you're inactive. Feeling sleepy is a sign that you have built up enough sleep power and your sleep rhythm is ready to let it loose. When you're fatigued or tired you may feel mentally or physically exhausted but be unable to fall asleep. If you're fatigued the best thing to do is wait to go to bed until you start to feel sleepy.

On the other hand, you might say that you never feel sleepy, that if you follow this power boost recommendation you'll never get to sleep. You're not alone. Many people with insomnia have a strained relationship with their sleepy self. You may feel as if you have completely lost touch with what it's like to feel sleepy. If this is true for you then you can choose to go to bed for any of the wrong reasons as long as you commit to following the sleep reprogramming techniques I talk about in Chapter 9. Over time, this will help you get back in touch with the feeling of sleepiness.

Power Boost #2: When to Get Up

When you get up in the morning can make a big difference. In fact, there are some of my colleagues who believe that this is the most important thing you could do to change your sleep pattern. Sleep is partly controlled by a powerful clock in the center of your brain. This makes time really important if you want great sleep. The simplest way to control the timing of sleep and sleep power is to get up at the same time every day. This will get your body into a nice sleep rhythm and when that happens...

- You maximize sleep power at bedtime, and

- Your brain can start to calculate exactly when to release that sleep power to put you to sleep.

Getting up at the same time each day is easier said than done. Especially for us night owls. Especially on the weekends. Especially after a difficult night. What's the best way to make getting up easier? Plan to do something you really love, something you can be excited about, first thing in the morning. Maybe it's exercise. Maybe it's a great cup of coffee or seeing the sunrise. Maybe it's getting together with a friend. Whatever you choose, this really can make it easier to maintain a consistent get up time. You may have to get creative and spend a little time planning this.

Power Boost #3: 8 hours or less in bed per night

It makes sense to spend more time in bed if you're having trouble sleeping. If you want to get eight hours and you know you're going to be up for two hours in the middle of the night then you should go to bed two hours earlier, right? Unfortunately, although the math works out to you getting eight hours of sleep, the real experience of insomnia doesn't play out that way. Spending more time in bed usually leads to lighter more broken sleep, without actually getting any more sleep than usual.

Because spending more time in bed makes so much sense and because it makes insomnia worse, most people with insomnia can benefit from this power boost. Here's how to do it. You almost certainly won't benefit from spending more than eight hours in bed so count back eight hours from the time you're choosing to get up each day. This will be the earliest time you will go to bed. If you're not sleepy at that time, then you'll wait until you are sleepy. But don't go to bed any earlier, even if you are sleepy.

That's the basic version. Now let's talk about the advanced version. Despite whatever horror stories you might have heard about sleep deprivation, mild sleep deprivation can be a very effective tool for boosting sleep power and providing rapid insomnia relief. For the advanced version, estimate how many hours of sleep you're getting per night on average. Five? Six? Seven? Whatever it is, add 30 minutes and then count back that many hours from the time you're choosing to get up each day. This is now your earliest bedtime. If you're not sleepy at that time then you'll wait until you are sleepy. But don't go to bed any earlier, even if you are sleepy. Try this for 14 days and you'll likely experience a meaningful shift in your sleep pattern and the quality of your sleep.

In addition to better sleep, there is also another bonus to trying the advanced version of this power boost. You magically create more time in your day. If you were spending 8 hours in bed per night and now you're planning to spend seven hours, you just gained an extra hour per day to do the things you've been complaining about not having time for. What will you do with this extra time each day?

Power Boost #4: Napping...or maybe not.

Remember how sleep power (adenosine) builds up in your brain every minute you're awake? Well, every minute you sleep, your sleep power is being drained away. This is why even a short nap in the late afternoon or evening can threaten your sleep at night.

When you nap it takes away from your sleep power at bedtime and can cause difficulty falling asleep, less sleep, and lighter more broken sleep. Because of this, it's best to avoid napping altogether. I know this can be difficult, especially after a poor night of sleep. It can help to think of the urge to nap like a craving. It will usually pass if you can distract yourself by doing something active for a few minutes.

With that said, sooner or later we all need a nap. In fact, if anyone ever tells you that you need a nap you're probably being a jerk and you should immediately get your blankie and find somewhere to lie down. But all joking aside, here's how you can use naps to get relief without ruining your sleep at night. I call these the "Sweet Nap" rules:

- Before you lie down, set an alarm for 30 minutes or less. When the alarm goes off, get up and go on with your day...even if you don't think you slept.

- If you're at home, it's best to nap in your bed. This helps build strong sleep programming. If you're away from home just be sure to choose a safe place. Many people like to lock the doors of their car and lay the seat back for a quick nap over lunch or before going home for the day.

- Finally, you absolutely want to avoid any napping or dozing within 6 hours of bedtime. Even 5-10 minutes of dozing while watching TV in the evening can cause difficulty falling asleep, lighter more restless sleep, and waking up too early.

Many people have a negative attitude about napping (only lazy people nap, right?). I think this is nonsense. Just seven to ten minutes of the lightest stage of sleep during a nap can provide up to three hours of benefit in terms of mood, alertness, and performance. So, I give you permission to take a short nap so you can spend your afternoons happy and productive, while those people who think napping is lazy spend their afternoons grouchy and spinning their wheels. Before I close this chapter, I'd like to speak to a few common concerns or objections to the Sweet Nap rules.

1. Many people complain that they could never even fall asleep in 30 minutes let alone get any actual rest during that time. Here's the thing. We humans are horrible at estimating when we fall asleep. This is partly because our minds can be active, thinking and aware of our surroundings, while the brain is in the lightest stages of sleep. So, chances are, you're getting beneficial sleep even if it doesn't feel the same as night time sleep.

2. Many people say they can't nap. Period. If you feel this way I would refer you to the previous bullet and add one thing. When it comes to naps, if you set aside the time to rest with the attitude of, "If I fall asleep, great! If I don't fall asleep, great!", you may be surprised to find yourself falling asleep unexpectedly or at least getting up from your "rest" period feeling better than you did when you laid down.

3. Many people complain that they need to sleep for at least an hour, maybe even two, for a nap to be worthwhile. I can understand that. I used to feel exactly that way. What I learned (and I'm so glad I did!) is that Sweet Naps are a learned skill, an acquired taste so to speak. It takes practice. If you commit to taking a Sweet Nap once a day for 14 days you will likely train your body to nap this way and you will probably like it. One more thing on long naps

versus Sweet Naps. Long naps are a problem because if you sleep for more than 30 minutes or so you're more likely to get into the deeper stages of sleep. Deeper sleep is much harder to wake up from, leaving you sluggish and groggy when you get up. Sweet Naps, however, give you a chance to get the restorative and refreshing benefit of lighter sleep, from which you can easily and quickly re-enter the flow of your day feeling great.

4. Many people say they don't have time to nap. That may be true for you. However, my experience is that most anyone who is motivated to make naps a consistent way of minimizing the effects of insomnia and maximizing performance seem to be able to successfully do so. Like anything else, time for naps can be found when they become a priority. If you need a little motivation, see my earlier comments about the boost in mood, alertness, and performance from as little as 10 minutes of light sleep.

Good Luck and Caution

That's it for the power boosts. Good luck getting started on these. One note of caution. Combined with insomnia, these power boost strategies can cause increased sleepiness in the daytime. Please remember that your safety and the safety of those around you is always the highest priority. Avoid driving or other activities that require optimal and sustained alertness and attention if you're feeling at all drowsy or foggy.

CHAPTER 9

LAW #6: INSOMNIA IS A PROGRAMMING PROBLEM

"...psychological and behavioral factors are ALMOST ALWAYS involved in perpetuating it [insomnia] over time."

– Charles Morin, World Renowned Insomnia Researcher[1]

What does he mean by "almost always"? Well, if you were to use the sleep transformation strategies that change these factors, there is a 90% chance you will get significantly better. Even more amazing, you would have a 40% chance of completely eliminating your insomnia. How can this be?

Experience of trouble sleeping over weeks or months actually changes your brain in a way that causes it to learn or become programmed to have trouble sleeping. Sometimes these changes are quite obvious and sometimes not so much. The most obvious signs your brain may be programmed for trouble sleeping are:

- You become wide awake, rather than sleepy, when you turn out the lights

- When you wake up in the night, you suddenly find yourself wide awake for no reason

- Thoughts and worries are waiting for you as soon as you wake in the night

- You sleep great when you're away from home on the couch, but in your own bed...it's just not happening

- You can't sleep even when you "should" be able to, like when you're sleep deprived, stress free, and had a physically demanding day

- Can't sleep without the TV on

Any one of these experiences may be a signal your brain has been programmed for insomnia. If you've had trouble sleeping for more than a few months, this insomnia programming has almost certainly become a part of the problem. What's worse, programmed insomnia happens no matter what started or may be perpetuating your trouble sleeping. Even if you have chronic pain that you know is causing you to sleep poorly, you almost certainly also have programmed insomnia. Even if you have sleep apnea that you know is causing you to sleep poorly, you almost certainly also have programmed insomnia. In fact, in a study published by my colleagues and me in the journal Sleep Medicine, over 50% of individuals with sleep apnea had insomnia that was separate from their breathing problem.[2] If you're still thinking you have some reason for not sleeping and that this idea of insomnia programming doesn't apply to you, go back and check out LAW #3: Insomnia Has a Life of Its Own (Chapter 6) again.

You May Find This Hard to Believe...

Most of you will have one of two common reactions to this idea of insomnia programming. The first reaction is that it makes perfect sense to you. If this is the case for you, you probably feel as if a glorious light is now shining down on your sleep problem. Finally, you clearly see what's going on and why your problem is so stubborn. Keep reading. It will get even clearer.

If you're not feeling this, then you're likely having the second common reaction, which involves the idea of insomnia programming sounding like complete nonsense or at least something fairly unbelievable that of course a psychologist would say.

That's okay. After working with literally hundreds of people with chronic insomnia I have found that the idea (and the power) of insomnia programming is probably the most misunderstood and difficult to believe laws of insomnia. This is unfortunate because it is likely the most important of the laws. It is also the law with the greatest promise for hope, power, and control over reclaiming your life and sleeping better again. Here's how it plays out in real life.

How Your Brain Gets Programmed for Insomnia in Five Steps

STEP 1.

IN THE BEGINNING...

The brain is programmed for sleep and connects the bed with feelings of calm, comfort, and sleepiness.

If you're like most people you probably remember a time when you slept well, when sleep was just something you enjoyed and didn't spend much time thinking about or trying to do. It just happened.

Even if you have been a light sleeper most of your life, your brain pretty much "knew what to do" when you got into bed.

STEP 2.

LIFE HAPPENS...

Stress or illness causes increased activation in your thoughts, emotions, and body, often in ways you may be unaware.

Just for this example, let's say you started having trouble sleeping because of stress. Maybe it was even good stress, like planning a wedding or starting a new job.

The specific stressor really doesn't matter – good stress, bad stress, injury, illness – any one or more of the "puzzle pieces" listed in Chapter 5 can start the process.

STEP 3.

INSOMNIA BEGINS...
Difficulty falling asleep, re-turning to sleep, or unrest-ful sleep become a regular experience, happening sev-eral nights per week. Maybe every night.

Aware of it or not, increased activation began to get in the way of your ability to sleep.

When you finally lay down you found your mind and body unready to let go and fall asleep. Instead, you found yourself lying there thinking or planning, uncomfortable, or maybe just too awake.

You may have started waking up more during the night. Instead of feeling drowsy and drifting quickly back to sleep, you woke up to full alertness and maybe even to a mind eager to think, plan, or worry.

Maybe you never actually got back to sleep, just woke up early and found yourself up for the rest of the day.

STEP 4.

THE BRAIN CHANGES...
Trouble sleeping many times over weeks or months causes changes in the brain.
The brain now connects the bed with being awake, worried, frustrated, or uncomfortable.

As the number of nights with troubled sleep stacks up and the consequences of poor sleep build, negative reactions and expectations around sleep take hold.

Over time, repeated experiences of frus-tration, wakefulness, restlessness, worry, or discomfort while in bed literally get you wired for insomnia.

Just as you're programmed for good feelings to come over you whenever you hear the first notes of your favorite song...

And just as you're programmed for feelings of sickness whenever you smell that food that made you so sick the last time you ate it...

You're now programmed for insomnia.

STEP 5.

PROGRAMMED FOR INSOMNIA...

The brain now connects the bed and bedroom with feelings of stress, activation, and sleeplessness.

You no longer need a reason to have trouble sleeping...it just happens.

Rather than being a place of calm, comfort, and sleepiness, your brain is now programmed to see your bed as an unpredictable and often unpleasant place where your hope for the blissful release of sleep is cruelly denied.

Insomnia now has a life of its own and you no longer need a reason to have trouble sleeping. Once this happens, your insomnia will continue even after the original reason for trouble sleeping is gone.

In order to return to a healthy satisfying sleep pattern, you will have to change the insomnia programming and reverse the brain changes. Sleep medications cannot do this.

Programmed for Insomnia

That last part is extremely important so I'm going to say it again. Once your brain learns to have trouble sleeping, once the insomnia programming has taken hold, unless you do something to change the program, you will continue to struggle even if you fix all other reasons for having insomnia. Insomnia programming works in your brain like a piece of software. The Free Dictionary has these two definitions of the word program that you may find interesting:

> *To train to perform automatically in a desired way, as if programming a machine: programmed the children to use perfect table manners.*

> *To inculcate [instill, saturate] with attitudes, behavior patterns, or the like; condition: to program children to respect their elders.*

Once the insomnia programming has been "installed" through repeated experiences of trouble sleeping and all the baggage that comes along with poor sleep, it works in just the way these definitions say. We can think of the insomnia program as malevolent and self-adapting.

Malevolent Program - a computer program designed to have undesirable or harmful effects

Self-Adapting Program - a program that can change its performance in response to its environment

Let's say you've had trouble sleeping for a few months or more and you're willing to believe that your brain has somehow been infected with this malevolent self-adapting insomnia program. NOW WHAT!?

No Worries – Installing a New Program is Simple

The behavioral technology for replacing a malevolent self-adapting insomnia program with a healthy sleep program has been around since the 1970's. Although challenging and somewhat unpleasant this reprogramming of the brain is relatively simple and can be done in a matter of about 14 days. Here's how:

Step 1: Escape the Bedroom

Get out of bed and go to another room if you're not asleep in 15-20 minutes. Every minute you lay in bed awake your brain is becoming more and more programmed for insomnia. This is why getting out of bed when you're unable to sleep is almost always the right thing to do.

Step 2: Hang Out

While you're out of bed, keep yourself occupied by doing something that is not activating - like watching TV, reading, or listening to music. You're not trying to make yourself sleepy, and you're not trying to be productive. You're literally just keeping yourself entertained without becoming too activated.

Step 3: Try Again

Go back to bed and try again after 15-20 minutes. You can think of this process of escaping the bedroom and hanging out as giving your brain a chance to "reset."

Step 4: Repeat

Follow steps 1-3 as many times as needed until you get into bed and fall asleep quickly.

This process of Escape, Hang Out, Try Again is unbelievably effective. In fact, if there was only one thing in this entire book you decide to actually do it should be this. It is so effective that this strategy and a couple of other related strategies are the primary sleep transformation tools used in the Sleep for Health, Healing, and Relapse Prevention (SHARP) program.

It is so important that I want to make sure you have access to the SHARP training video that teaches these tools. Go to www.coloradoinsomni-aclinic.com/sharpsleeptraining and you will have free access to the video. It is just under 30 minutes long and the sooner you watch it the sooner you will know how to hack that malevolent self-adapting insomnia program out of your brain.

Rapid Insomnia Relief

When you combine the power boosts, the Escape, Hang Out, Try Again process, and other strategies in the SHARP training you have everything you need to create radical sleep transformation in a matter of 14-21 days.

PART 3

RADICAL SLEEP TRANSFORMATION™:
ADVANCED INSOMNIA RELIEF

CHAPTER 10

LAW #7: INSOMNIA IS A MIND PROBLEM

"Insomnia can be caused by responding to an acute normal episode of insomnia by interpreting it as a sign of danger or loss of control and beginning to monitor sleep loss and worry about its consequences."

Charles Morin and Colin Espie[1]

Have you ever thought, "If only I could learn to turn my mind off, I would sleep just fine?" One of the most frustrating things about insomnia for many people is the experience of being unable to sleep because they're unable to turn off their thoughts. This is easy to understand when your mind is stuck on important things. It's especially maddening when the thoughts you're stuck on seem completely meaningless or insignificant.

The way we think and what we believe about sleep and insomnia affects every aspect of insomnia. Because of this, you will notice that some of the things I talk about in this chapter overlap with what I've said in other chapters. No, I'm not crazy. These things really are that important.

No, It's not All In Your HEAD (Well...maybe a little.)

Thoughts have a powerful effect on sleep. Here's an example. Let's say you heard a news story that said terrible things will happen if you don't get 8 hours of sleep a night. If you take this seriously then you might begin pay-ing much closer attention to your sleep patterns and habits. If you began trying to get 8 hours but for some reason can only get 7, you might start putting a lot of energy into figuring out how to get 8 hours. You might start to worry about what's wrong with you that your body won't let you get 8 hours. You might then worry about what this means. If you're not getting 8 hours then maybe all those terrible things are going to happen to you. Now the pressure to sleep, the worry about not sleeping as much as you think you should, and the worry about the consequences of this set the stage for you to become programmed for insomnia. In this example, the negative thinking pattern around sleep started because of a belief about sleep that caused worry even though there was no actual sleep problem. Imagine how the mind can get worked up when faced with real repeated sleeplessness.

Sleep Worry: Twisted Beliefs and Expectations about Sleep

Although stress can cause increased worry both at bedtime and when you wake up at night (I'll talk more about that in Chapter 13), your mind really doesn't need any stress to get worked up and refuse to shut down for sleep. Your beliefs and expectations about sleep and the consequences of sleep loss can actually cause and perpetuate insomnia. In fact, sometimes all it takes for your mind to start a cycle of chronic insomnia are some troubling thoughts about why you're not sleeping and what will happen if you don't. Whatever your situation, in most cases, these five types of think-ing problems cause or worsen insomnia:[1]

- Beliefs about the cause of insomnia that lead to feelings of help-lessness or inaction

- Catastrophic thoughts about what insomnia is doing to you, your life, or your body

- Expectation for "Supernatural Sleep"

- Feeling and thinking your sleep is under the control of some mysterious force

- Beliefs about fixing insomnia that actually make insomnia worse

Beliefs about the Causes of Insomnia

Your beliefs about why you have insomnia fundamentally drive what you decide to do about it. In fact, these beliefs essentially define what you think you're able to do about insomnia. There is a longer discussion of this issue In Chapter 6 (LAW #3: Insomnia Has a Life of Its Own). Sooner or later most people with insomnia try to come up with an explanation for why they have insomnia and why the things they have tried to fix the insomnia have not worked. Often, the explanation is something that is thought to be out of one's control. This might be the belief that a chemical imbalance, medical illness, mental illness, stress, or some other factor is the primary cause of the sleep problem.

These things may certainly be contributing to the sleep problem. However, unless they are severe and untreated, they are almost certainly not the only thing (or even the main thing) causing your insomnia. In Chapter 5 (LAW #2: Insomnia Has Many Causes) I talked about the puzzle of poor sleep and how most sleep problems are caused by more than one thing. In Chapter 6 (LAW #3: Insomnia Has a Life of Its Own) I talked about how insomnia is often independent of other health problems and in Chapter 9 (LAW #6: Insomnia is a Programming Problem) I talked about how almost every person who experiences chronic insomnia becomes programmed to have trouble sleeping. For all of these reasons, any belief that blames insomnia on a single cause is likely incorrect and risks leading you down a road to helplessness and hopelessness. A brilliant insomnia researcher named Art Spielman came up with a beautiful explanation of this called the 3 P's. There's no room to go into it here. But, if you want to really understand how the causes of insomnia interact and change over time, check out this free online article: http://www.med.upenn.edu/psychotherapy/user_documents/CausesofInsomnia.[2]

Catastrophic Thoughts about What Insomnia Is Doing To You

Although lying awake at night may be lonely, boring or even miserable, it's probably not what leads you to read this book and it's not what leads most people with insomnia to seek help. What really fills The Insomnia Clinic and drives big drug company profits is the fear that not sleeping will drive you crazy, destroy your body, or otherwise ruin your life. Fear of the consequences of sleep loss can be intense, so intense that this fear can turn into the cause of insomnia fairly quickly.

Now, don't get me wrong, insomnia is a big deal and chronic sleep loss can take its toll on our bodies, minds, and relationships. However, the actual effect of insomnia in our lives is rarely as tragic as our fears would have us believe. Maybe you worry that you're always irritable because of your insomnia and this brings on thoughts like, "My wife is going to leave me and my kids are going to hate me because I'm such a grouch." Maybe you worry you will make a mistake at work and this worry brings on thoughts like, "It's just a matter of time before I lose my job" or "I could really hurt someone." Maybe you worry you won't be able to think clearly or speak intelligently and this brings on thoughts like," People will think I'm stupid."

Think about your own experience. Take a moment and bring to mind three negative thoughts you have had about what will happen if you don't get enough sleep. All of these things are possible. No doubt. But...they are also highly unlikely. Now think about how many nights you've had insomnia. Hundreds? Thousands? With this in mind, how many times have the tragic things you fear actually happened? If you are like most of us who have suffered with insomnia, the horrible things we fear rarely, if ever, actually come to pass.

Finally, it may make you feel somewhat better to know you are probably getting more sleep than you think. The sleep centers are connected to the memory centers and trying to remember anything around sleep can be a challenge. Because of this, we almost universally underestimate the amount of sleep we get. One thing that happens after having insomnia for a while is that our estimates of sleep get even more distorted. This is one reason why many people with insomnia are surprised at how well they function during the day despite what seems like major sleep loss. Bottom line? Even though the sleep may be poor or not enough, you're probably getting enough to meet your body's most basic needs. This is why the most significant health effects connected to insomnia occur only in those who sleep less than 5 hours per night as recorded in a sleep laboratory.

Expectation for Supernatural Sleep

What is normal sleep? What does it look like? What does it feel like? With the exception of what we hear in the media or from family or friends, most of us get no information about what "normal" sleep actually looks like. This sets the stage for negative thoughts and reaction to "normal" nights of poor sleep. So what is normal sleep? As we age, sleep tends to become lighter and more broken up. However, as older adults, we still need about the same amount of sleep to feel and function well as we did in our twenties. Most people need between seven and nine hours of sleep per night. Taking up to 30 minutes to fall asleep and spending up to 30 minutes awake during the night is considered normal. Waking up one or two times during the night is also normal.

It is also normal for your sleep pattern to fluctuate from night to night. Maybe last night you fell asleep in 5 minutes and slept until your alarm went off. Maybe tonight you'll lie in bed for 25 minutes before falling asleep and then wake up for 10 minutes at 3 am. Both experiences would be considered normal. The more you can go with the flow of night-to-night changes in sleep the less chance your mind will have to cause insomnia.

This reality that natural sleep can be better or worse from one night to the next can be problematic once a person is on sleeping pills and wants to stop using them. In some cases sleeping pills can produce sleep that is more consistent and more satisfying than natural sleep. If you've had this experience then you may find it takes some time to adjust to normal sleep after stopping a sleeping pill.

Out of Control and Powerless in the Face of Some Mysterious Force

Repeated experiences of sleeplessness can quickly lead to feelings of being out of control. In fact, it's not uncommon to feel as if your sleep is under the influence of some mysterious force over which you have no control. This often leads to "performance anxiety." Worried about your inability to sleep, you begin to try harder to make sleep happen by developing specific, even very precise and lengthy evening or bedtime routines, in an attempt to control sleep. Unfortunately, as you well know if you've been in this situation, the harder you try to sleep, the harder it is.

In the face of this frustrating reality it can be useful to take an "opposite action" approach. If you can't sleep and nothing you do seems to help you regain control, then maybe the best thing to do is stop trying to sleep altogether. Don't go to bed until you start falling asleep on the couch watching TV. If you get into bed and find yourself wide awake, go with it. Plan to keep your eyes open and stay awake as long as you can. If sleep still doesn't come then you're really no worse off then you were when you were trying so hard to make it happen. If sleep sneaks up on you and you accidentally fall asleep, great! You can be grateful for whatever sleep you got. As a side note, just FYI, a good bedtime routine should be no more than 20 minutes long and should result in you being able to progressively relax and unwind.

Even if you don't fall into this trap of performance anxiety and trying too hard to sleep, it can be quite nerve wracking to feel like difficulties sleeping are happening for no reason. Don't be fooled. It may seem like insomnia comes out of nowhere, but if you look closely there is almost always some reason for a night of poor sleep. It can be helpful to spend a few minutes taking an honest and critical look at the day or so leading up to a bad night of sleep. Take a look at Chapter 12 (LAW #9: It's a 24-Hour Problem) for ideas about how to do this and what to look for.

Finally, after a while it can feel like insomnia is taking over your life. You may find yourself thinking about your sleep problem day and night. You may find yourself changing plans when you've had a bad night of sleep.

You may start avoiding things that you fear may make you more activated and make your sleep problem worse. If you start worrying about sleep all the time and shaping your day-to-day activities around your sleep problem, sooner or later you will find that your life has begun to shrink around you. Don't let this happen. If it has already begun to happen, understand you are not helpless. You can change this. Although insomnia steals energy, motivation and interest, you are still the one that gets to choose what you do each and every hour of every day. As with performance anxiety, it can often be useful to take an "opposite action" approach or an "as if I wasn't _____" (sleep deprived, fatigued, grumpy) attitude. From this perspective you will experiment with acting as if you had not had a poor night of sleep. How would go through your day if you had slept well and weren't fatigued or mentally foggy?

Beliefs about Fixing Insomnia

When it comes to fixing insomnia and responding to a poor night of sleep, what "makes sense" often makes the problem worse. Because of this, the thoughts and beliefs you have about fixing insomnia significantly influence your ability to take action that moves you toward better sleep. These thoughts and beliefs about fixing insomnia are so influential that I've dedicated the majority of two chapters of this book to them. Rather than repeat that information here, I encourage you to read Chapter 6 (LAW #3: Insomnia has a Life of Its Own) and Chapter 7 (LAW #4: Insomnia is a Tricky Problem). The information in these chapters will help you to get rid of old beliefs that lead you to do things that make insomnia worse. The most common ones are:

- If I don't get enough sleep, I need to make up for it by staying in bed longer, napping, or going to bed early.

- When I have trouble sleeping, I should stay in bed and try harder.

- As long as I spend enough time in bed I'll get the sleep I need.

The Vicious Cycle

Now that you know the primary kinds of thinking problems connected to insomnia, it's important to know how thoughts work. Our thoughts are powerful in several ways and our thoughts interact with our body and emotions to create a cycle that starts insomnia, and perpetuates it long term.

The Mind Problem Part 1

Thoughts are like rabbits. Whether positive or negative, they breed fast. A negative thought about sleep or the consequences of not sleeping leads to more negative thoughts, which lead to even more negative thoughts, ultimately turning into a spiral of negative thinking that often leads to the "death of sleep."

As if the thoughts themselves weren't enough, our thoughts, beliefs, and emotions change our body. A series of negative thoughts almost universally leads to muscle tension, increased heart rate, higher blood pressure, and many other changes in the body in the direction of activation or what is sometimes called hyperarousal (or even agitation). Needless to say, activation and agitation in the mind or body is the enemy of sleep.

The Mind Problem Part 2

Once a pattern of negative thinking (thoughts, beliefs, expectations) and hyperarousal around sleep begins, it will start to "feed" on itself. Whereas good sleepers rarely think about sleep, insomniacs often find themselves worrying about sleep and the consequences of insomnia. Thoughts and worries about sleep may begin early in the evening or even during the day. This causes more activation or hyperarousal in the body and emotions. Hyperarousal at bedtime then fuels increased worry about the ability to sleep, and more difficulty sleeping. Ultimately, the thoughts about sleep become connected to the bed and bedroom (see Chapter 9 about sleep programming) and the body and mind turn on rather than off when you want to sleep.

Taking Control of Your Mind

This is all fascinating, but how do you actually break this pattern? There are a variety of ways. The most common recommendation is "worry time," which basically means taking time each evening to empty your mind of thoughts or worries by journaling. Theoretically, this will keep you from taking the troublesome thoughts to bed with you. Distraction techniques like counting sheep or counting backwards by 3's are also frequently recommended. These can sometimes work but most people I talk to don't find them very helpful.

The most effective way to actually break the cycle of thoughts and drain the power out of the negative thoughts, beliefs, and expectations is to directly confront them with a three step process of "identify, examine/challenge, and rethink." Here's how:

Identify

Write down your thoughts and beliefs about sleep. It is best to keep something with you to take notes throughout the day. Once you start paying attention to what your mind is doing, you may be surprised at when and how often thoughts about sleep come up. You can download a questionnaire designed to help identify common thinking problems of insomnia here:[3]

http://www.fss.ulaval.ca/cms_recherche/upload/chaire_sommeil/fichiers/dysfunctional_beliefs_and_attitudes_about_sleep__30_items.pdf

Examine/Challenge

Once you have a list of the thoughts you're having about your sleep or the consequence of your sleep problem, it's time to take a close look at them. Here are some questions you might ask yourself as you begin to examine your thoughts:

- Is this really true?

- What facts support this thought?

- What is the evidence against this thought?

- Is there a better explanation for what's happening?

- What's the worst that could happen? Could I handle it?

- What's the best that could happen?

- What's the most realistic thing that could happen?

- What would I tell a friend if they were having the same problem?

- How would someone else see my situation?

Rethink

Once you've had a chance to take a close look at the thoughts and beliefs, take a little time to write down alternative thoughts/beliefs that are more true or accurate than the original automatic thoughts. Then when the old automatic thoughts come up, you'll have more accurate, useful, and less distressing thoughts to replace them with.

Conclusion

Which of the five types of thinking problems do you recognize? Now that you understand how thoughts and beliefs about sleep "kick start" the vicious cycle of negative thoughts and hyperarousal, it's critical to take control of your mind. Begin using the three steps of Identify, Challenge, and Rethink to shut down the cycle and begin to see sleep and insomnia in a new, healthier way.

CHAPTER 11

LAW #8: SLEEP IS SLIPPERY

Insomnia can be controlled, but sleep can't. Sleep is one of those squirrely things that is harder to do the more you chase after it. In fact, I think of sleep as the ridiculous art of doing nothing. While you sleep, your mind and body are busy doing the amazing work of replenishing and restoring you in every way...but your job is to do nothing.

Unfortunately, most of us are downright horrible at doing nothing. Doing nothing requires us to let go of all the things we have to keep control over during the day. This is easier said than done.

"Just let go." Yeah right!

The harder you try to sleep, the harder it is to get. Has anyone ever told you something like this? "Sleep is easy. You just let go." I've actually had a person, let's call him Martin, say to me, yelling, "How do I do that?! What does that even mean!?" This is when it really struck me how ridiculous this statement is, especially if it is not followed up with some concrete way of actually doing it.

I didn't get upset with Martin. He was genuinely struggling to fix his sleep problem. He was working hard to follow the recommendations I had given him to that point. As we were talking that particular day I realized he was trying too hard. He was desperate to get more sleep. It was like he was wrestling a greased pig. Huffing and puffing, chasing sleep around the house at night. Anytime he got close to it, it would just slip away. Sooner or later he got exhausted enough to just give up. As soon as he gave up, as soon as he resigned himself to not sleeping that night, he would find that tricky old pig snuggled right up to him and he would drift off to sleep.

Unbelievable, right? Well, not so much. This happens all the time in many areas of life. It came up recently with my wife and mother. They are both addicted to this puzzle game called Candy Crush. Maybe you've heard of it? Only like a million people play it. It was Father's Day and we were all sitting around after our meal and I hear my wife complaining about how she had been on level 2000 or something for weeks. She had been playing every night for about an hour before bed (not recommended but she sleeps like a baby so I don't complain). Then my mother chimed in; she too had been stuck. They started talking about how they tried to solve the puzzle of this level. She had seen the solutions on Google from the experts and tried those. They were really frustrated that they had put so much time and effort into this game and seemed to be getting nowhere. They seemed to get some catharsis from sharing their frustration but that was about it.

About two weeks later my mom said to my wife excitedly, "I did it! I solved that level!" "How?" my wife asked. "I just said screw it. I was so frustrated I just started playing like I didn't even care," my mother responded. "Next thing I knew I was through it." My wife was begrudgingly happy for her; she was still on level 2000 with no hope in sight.

You've probably heard similar stories in golf and other sports or in various creative pursuits. Another way it is said is, "You can't focus on the goal. Stay focused on the present and the goal will create itself." Sounds like nonsense, but somehow it works.

Now, my mother's success involved a video game. I know that games are important to people. I am a gamer myself and have thrown a controller or two in my time. But I think we can all agree that a sleep problem has a bit higher stakes. It hard to just say screw it and approach sleep like you just don't care. You do care and if you say you don't then you are probably just lying to yourself. Rather than say you don't care, it can be easier to play hard to get.

Your sleep wants you too, but sometimes you have to play hard to get

"Just let go of your worry about sleeping." "Just let go of your fear of what will happen if you don't sleep." Although easier said than done, this is exactly what's needed - to act like you don't care if you sleep or not. When you're playing hard to get, you do care about the thing that you want but are resisting it in order to build tension and suspense and excitement. There is some fun, even exhilaration, in toying and teasing. So, what does this look like? How do you "play hard to get" with sleep? Here's the four step process:

Invite Sleep:

You do this in two ways. First, you need to act like you want sleep to come and hang out with you. This means that you need to have a calming bedtime routine that you follow each night for about 20 minutes before you plan to turn out the lights. Second, you have to actually turn out the lights and lie down intending and expecting to sleep.

Observe the Reaction:

Now that you've invited sleep to come, what happens? Does sleep accept your invitation, allowing you to fall asleep easily? Or, is sleep just not that into you? You've made the invitation, now it's time to watch what happens. Just know that the less interested you seem the more desirable you become.

Play it Cool:

Whatever happens, relax and let it happen. Do you feel drowsy? Tense? Relaxed? Worried? Frustrated? Peaceful but awake? Just watch whatever is going on with a sense of passive curiosity. You're saying to sleep, "If you want to hang out, that's cool." This is very different than the automatic reaction that's usually something like, "Please. What do I have to do to for you to hang out with me? I'll do anything! I can't live without you!"

Turn Away:

You can't wait forever. You've made the invitation and you've given sleep a chance to see how awesome you are. If sleep does not come after 15 minutes or so, you simply say to yourself, "Oh, well. Sleep must not be ready yet. I'll just go do something else for a while and see if it wants to hang out a little later." Remember, sleep wants you too! As long as you can keep cool and not seem too desperate, sooner or later sleep will accept your invitation and you'll find yourself having the night of your life.

Summary

Sound ridiculous? Maybe. But research has shown that taking this passive approach to trouble sleeping actually works. Whatever you think about it, if what you're doing now isn't working, what do you have to lose? Playing hard to get is largely a mind game. As you know if you've struggled with insomnia for any length of time, insomnia can really do a number on you psychologically. This is the focus of Chapter 10 (LAW #7: Insomnia is a Mind Problem). It's also a 24-hour problem, which is the focus of the next chapter.

CHAPTER 12

LAW #9: INSOMNIA IS A 24-HOUR PROBLEM

One major limitation to people finding the right solution to their insomnia problem is a belief that insomnia is exclusively a nighttime problem. In reality, how you sleep at night is dramatically influenced by everything you do throughout the day and evening hours.

Circadian Rhythm (The Body Clock)

There is a little group of cells in the center of your brain called the suprachiasmatic nucleus. This tiny group of cells is your body's clock. It controls the circadian rhythm or timing for activity in every cell of your body throughout the 24-hour day. This includes the timing of when your brain and body are ready and willing to fall asleep and wake up. If you try to go to sleep when your body clock wants to be awake it can be near impossible. At the other end, trying to wake up when your body clock wants to be asleep can be like pulling teeth. With this in mind, it is critical to create a sleep schedule that is in line with your body's internal timing. A schedule that is out of alignment with the internal clock is a sure recipe for insomnia and daytime/evening sleepiness in a variety of forms. In addition to choosing a schedule that agrees with your clock, it's also important to understand how your activity during the day can change or reset your clock.

Specific activities that influence the body clock include bright light (including light from screens like those on phones, tablets, and computers) and timing of meals and exercise.

The Clock and The Insomnia Clinic

When you come to the clinic we take the time to look at your sleep problems from this 24-hour perspective. We start to look at possible contributors to your sleep problem throughout every part of the 24-hour day. Similarly, we also look for solutions throughout every part of the day.

- Do we need to negotiate a new bedtime or evening routine?

- Do we need to strategize changes to your napping pattern so you can get relief from sleepiness and fatigue during the day without ruining your sleep at night?

- How can we balance work, family, and fun in a way that gives you time to live your best life while getting you the sleep you need so you can love every minute you spend living it?

These are the kinds of questions that create an understanding of how your insomnia fits into your life throughout the 24-hour day and how to maximize sleep and life satisfaction. It can be helpful in the big picture of figuring out the causes and solutions for your insomnia. It can also help by reducing the mystery and frustration that are often connected to any single bad night of sleep. You can use the exercise below to find general causes of insomnia that affect your sleep on a regular basis. You can also use it to help figure out causes of insomnia after a specific night of poor sleep.

24-Hour Activity and Experience Exercise

The purpose of this exercise is to take a look at your day-to-day experiences and activities and make an honest judgment about their effect on the quality of your sleep and your ability to get to sleep and stay asleep. Keep in mind that the effects of day and evening activities and experiences on your sleep may not be obvious. Also, your beliefs about what "should" or "should not" influence your sleep can get in the way of figuring out what's really important. As best you can, set aside any preconceived ideas or assumptions about what may be influencing your sleep when you go through this exercise. Use the 24-Hour Activity and Experience Tracker at the end of this chapter to "walk through" your day from the time you wake up in the morning until you begin trying to sleep.

Step 1. Write down what you're doing and the time you are doing it.

Use columns one and two to track your activities and experiences throughout the day. It's best to do this at least once an hour, more if you're frequently changing activities or you have a particularly important experience. However, you can complete this at the end of the day if you don't have time throughout the day to be tracking your activities.

You may be wondering what exactly you should be putting on the tracker. You want to make frequent enough entries on the tracker to have a good sense of the variety of activities and flow of your day when you take time to look back at it at the end of the day. With that said, you will want to track all of the routine activities (driving to work, making dinner) you're involved in throughout the day, as well as any significant or unusual activities or experiences (argument with family member, bad or good news at work). There is no need to describe the activity in any detail. The entry on the tracker is only to help you remember the activity for steps two and three.

Step 2. Rate your belief about the effect of this activity or experience on your sleep.

In the third column enter a plus sign (+) if you think the effect of the activity or experience is positive or helpful. Enter a negative sign (-) if it is unhelpful. Enter a zero (0) if you feel the activity or experience is neutral or has no effect on your sleep. As you choose a rating, take a few moments to get a sense of your physical body, emotional experience, and thinking patterns while involved in each item you put on the tracker sheet. You can use the fourth column to enter any thoughts or insights you have about the effect of a specific activity or experience on your sleep.

Step 3. Look for patterns of activity or experience that may be influencing your sleep.

At the end of the day spend some time looking at the pattern of activity and experience throughout the day and evening hours. Some common patterns that can strongly influence your sleep include:

- Intense pleasant or unpleasant emotional experiences within 1-2 hours of bedtime

- "non-stop" activity or "busyness" right up until bedtime

- Intentional or unintentional dozing in the evenings

- Moderate to high intensity exercise too close to bedtime or after waking up too early

- Inadequate rest or recovery opportunity throughout the day

- Frequent moderate to high stress or chronic mild stress

Step 4. Connect your activity and experience patterns to your good and poor sleep on sleep logs.

The 24-Hour Activity and Experience Tracker can be extremely helpful when used in conjunction with sleep logs. I haven't talked about sleep logs in this book but they are an excellent way to track sleep patterns. If you've been keeping sleep logs, then you may want to begin to compare your day-to-day activities and experiences to your actual sleep patterns. Doing this can help to connect specific activities or experiences directly to nights of good or poor sleep.

Step 5. Do more of what improves sleep and less of what makes it worse.

It's fairly likely that you will come away from this exercise with some specific ideas about what strengthens your sleep and what breaks it down. It's time to come up with a plan. How will you begin to do more of the things you believe strengthen sleep? How will you eliminate the things you think are getting in the way?

Rest-Activity Patterns

Here are some things to think about as you go through this exercise:

Exercise patterns and habits:

- When do you exercise?

- How often, how long, and how intensely do you exercise?

- What are your body's natural rest and activity patterns?

Natural energy patterns:

- When do you feel energetic and inspired?

- When do you feel tired and worn down?

- When do you nap, and for how long?

Your approach to sleep:

- Do you come at bedtime running full speed, expecting to go from "zoom to stop?"

- Do you have a relaxing bedtime routine?

- If you have one, how long is your bedtime routine?

Your emotional experience throughout the day and evening:

- Was it a good day at work or did they announce layoffs?

- Did you have a wonderful conversation with your family before bed or was it an argument?

- Were you rushed and stressed all day or did you have a fairly leisurely day?

Other things to consider:

- When and what do you eat and drink?

- What is the latest you have caffeine, alcohol, or nicotine?

- How much sunlight do you get during the day and when?

Conclusion

Taking this 24-hour perspective on your insomnia has the potential to uncover sources of trouble sleeping that may surprise you. Complete the 24-hour Activity and Experience exercise with an open and honest attitude. This exercise can also help you begin to see potential sources of stress that are the focus of the next chapter.

SLEEP TRANSFORMATION:
24-HOUR ACTIVITY AND EXPERIENCE TRACKER

Time	Activity/Experience	Effect on Sleep (+ o -)	Notes/Thoughts

CHAPTER 13

LAW #10: INSOMNIA IS A STRESS PROBLEM

If you're Not Stressed You're Dead. Whether by good stress or bad stress, whether we are aware of it or not, we are all stressed. The real question is: are you willing to admit it? Even under some of the most troubling circumstances I find that people have a tendency to minimize their level of stress either by dismissing it, "My life is great. I really don't have any reason to be stressed," or by minimizing it, "Yes, caring for my ailing parents is challenging, but it's not like I'm living in a war zone." The bottom line is that Stress is our default state, the inevitable reality of the human experience. In most cases, we adapt and overcome. Other times we may be unable to adjust because the stress is too chronic, intense, or unpredictable. This is when stress can have an even more significant effect. Accordingly, stress is commonly an important part of insomnia, especially when it's a constant part of life.

Your sleep problem may be a stress problem

If you have trouble sleeping and nothing you do seems to help, these little known types of stress may be silently wreaking havoc on your sleep. To understand why these kinds of stress are an almost universal problem, let's start with a few hard facts about sleep:

- Sleep is a stationary activity.

- Sleep requires you to set aside the concerns of the day.

- Sleep is not something you do, but something that happens to you.

This means that if we want to sleep well and consistently we must...stop...let go...and let it happen.

This is a problem because of six kinds of stress

Going Stress

More and more we spend our days pushing ourselves full speed, morning to night. If you are a "normal" American this is how your day might look:

Wake up > rush out the door > Go. Go. Go. > Have a free moment, but decide to fill it with something like email, Facebook, chores or phone calls > Go some more > Skip lunch or at least keep going while you eat > Go. Go. Go. > Maybe have dinner, but don't stop now or you might not get started again so Go. Go. Go. > Get in bed and try to sleep.

After going like this day after day you will forget how to stop. You will forget how to be still while awake. If you forget how to be still while awake, you can no longer stop long enough for sleep to take you.

Tangle Stress

Sleep is supposed to be an escape, an opportunity for you to recharge and recover in a way that allows you to meet the next day feeling refreshed and renewed. In order for this to happen you must be able to let go of the pressures and worries of the day for a little while. This is difficult because you likely have so many things going on and so much to keep track of with your mind that it's almost impossible to let it all go. Everything you want to, have to, need to, would like to, forgot to, should, or must DO creates what's called an open loop.[1]

Open loops create mental and physical tension that lasts until you "close" the loops by doing whatever it is you need to do. Every open loop creates tension, no matter how small or unimportant it may seem. You probably have dozens (maybe more) of these open loops at the end of any given day.

What happens to your open loops when bedtime comes? Well, you may juggle your loops skillfully, gracefully, and joyfully throughout the day and then set them aside so you can sleep blissfully most nights. More likely, you get tangled up in the tension of these loops and find you can't get untangled when bedtime arrives. If you get too used to the tangle, you may forget that this tangle stress is even there. Once this happens, you won't "feel" stressed, but the tension of your open loops will leave you awake and wondering why you can't sleep.

Control Stress

Sleep is one of those things that becomes harder to get the more you try to get it. It's something that happens to you, something you have to let happen rather than something you do. Unfortunately, most of us are not that good at just letting things happen...even when we really, really want to.

When was the last time you thought, "Oooh, I'm hungry. Let me just relax here a while. I'm sure something yummy will come along."? The whole idea of sitting still and doing nothing when you really want or need something (like sleep) goes against our every instinct. Unfortunately, this is exactly how sleep works. This issue of being unable to control sleep is the entire focus of Chapter 11 (LAW #8: Sleep is Slippery), so I'm not going to get into it any deeper here.

Thinking Stress

We've all experienced a time when trying to sleep and can't seem to stop thinking about something that happened during the day, something coming up tomorrow or some stress in our life. These thoughts that arise when things get still, and dark, and quiet at night can be a good indicator of stress in our lives.

Maybe you're facing pressure at work. Maybe you're planning a wedding or expecting a baby. Maybe you've had an argument with someone close to you. Whatever it is, "losing sleep over it," is normal if whatever it is you're thinking about is important to you. You're supposed to think, and plan, and worry about these things to some degree, and its normal for this activity of your mind to override the sleep system for a time. When the stressful thing passes, your mind calms down and you're able to sleep again...at least that's how it's supposed to work. But what happens when you get into a worry habit and your mind continues to try to problem solve the things that are stressing you out? Well, unless you're taking steps during the day to choose and direct the attention and content of your mind then there is no reason to expect you'll be able to direct your thoughts away from stress when you want to at bedtime. Take a look at Chapter 10 (LAW #7: Insomnia is a Mind Problem) for more on how your mind may be fueling the fires of insomnia.

Relationship Stress

Good, bad, or ugly, our relationships with others are almost always the most important aspect of our lives. Whether with our parents or our children, our partners or friends, our coworkers, employees or bosses, our relationships affect us for better or worse. These effects happen whether we like it or not. In his book *Social Intelligence*, Daniel Goleman talks about two aspects of relationship that can't help but affect our sleep.[2]

Emotional Contagion and Mirror Neurons

"At an unconscious level, we are in constant dialogue with anyone we interact with, our every feeling and very way of moving attuned to theirs."[2]

Emotions are contagious. We don't just sense what others are feeling we actually "mirror" what they are feeling in our own brains and bodies. In order to understand the situation and the relationship fully we actually take on the emotional experience of the other person at the most basic physical and neurological level. This has powerful implications for our ability to sleep.

If the people around us are happy and friendly and calm at bedtime we will have that experience as we prepare for bed and lie down to sleep. If the people around us are stressed, frustrated, upset, or angry at bedtime, then we may basically be "sleeping with the enemy" as our emotional state is likely to infect us with those anti-sleep emotions.

Rehashing Relationships

> *"...the brain's default activity – what happens when nothing much else goes on – seems to be mulling over our relationships."*[2]

If our relationships are great then this background rehashing of our relationships probably creates a sense of calm and security that is likely to promote sleep. However, if our relationships are in conflict this rehashing may significantly interfere with the winding down and letting go necessary to initiate sleep. This aspect of relationship stress is particularly important in relationships characterized by chronic conflict or dissatisfaction, especially when those relationships are with a spouse, partner, or child.

Regret and Guilt Stress

Regret and guilt stress are related to tangle stress but they're common enough and have a big enough effect on our level of stress, I like to talk about them separately. Remember that tangle stress is caused by open loops, which create mental and physical tension that lasts until you "close" the loops by taking some action to finalize or resolve them.

A normal open loop involves anything and everything you want to, have to, need to, would like to, forgot to, should, or must DO that is left unresolved at the end of the day. Open loops due to regret or guilt involve things we have done or failed to do that we are not proud of or wish we had handled differently. Depending on the incident, these open loops may have stronger or weaker effects on our level of stress and sleep.

Regret and guilt stress are a unique problem because we tend to avoid closing the loops they create. Think about it. We all do things we are not proud of pretty much every day. We say things to the people we care about that are hurtful or speak to them in a hurtful tone. We cut someone off in traffic or behave rudely because we are in a hurry. We all say and do things with the potential to open loops of guilt or regret, even if not intentionally. Pretty much anything we do that does not fit with our sense of integrity can cause these types of open loops. Not doing the things we know we need to do to take care of ourselves is another good example. "I should spend more time playing with the kids." Or, "I need to be going to the gym and not eat so many sweets."

Now think about the last time you took action to resolve these types of open loops. When was the last time you apologized? When was the last time you actively caught yourself not doing something you thought you should, and then made a choice to change your behavior in that direction? If your answer is "not recently" or "not very often" then welcome to the club. Because these loops are connected with feelings of guilt or regret, they can be particularly hard to close. This is why they can lurk in the background causing unrecognized stress for long periods of time.

What to do? Mindfulness-Based Meditation

There are many ways to handle stress but I have developed a particular liking for mindfulness training. Mindfulness based meditation is emerging as one of the most powerful ways to manage both sleep and stress problems. In fact, mindfulness recently made the cover of Time magazine.[3] Science is also proving the power of mindfulness for better sleep. In one study, mindfulness based meditation was compared to the sleep drug Lunesta for treatment of insomnia.[4] The researchers in this study found that meditation resulted in sleep improvements equal to those obtained with medication - the difference of course being the lack of dependence or dangerous side effects associated with meditation. Another group of researchers from Stanford University combined mindfulness based meditation with sleep transformation training. They found that this combined strategy helped participants significantly reduce sleep effort and pre-sleep arousal, two factors associated with insomnia.[5] These benefits were mostly maintained a year after the end of the study.[6]

Mindfulness meditation can eliminate all kinds of stress. Here's how...

- Forgoing stress, mindfulness helps you relearn how to be still while awake, helping you stop and set the stage for sleep.

- For tangle stress, mindfulness teaches you how to see and untangle your tangles, or at least leave the tangled mess out in the kitchen until the next morning, so you can get a good night's sleep.

- For control stress, mindfulness supports learning to be patient and comfortable with allowing things to unfold in their own time, helping you become an expert at letting sleep happen.

- For thinking stress, mindfulness cultivates the ability to choose the direction of your attention so you'll be able to direct your thoughts away from stress at bedtime.

- For relationship stress, mindfulness helps you become more aware of tension and stress in the relationships with those most important to you. It also helps you to begin to change the effect of contagious emotions on your sleep.

- For regret and guilt stress, mindfulness encourages you to see your actions without judgment; this takes the sting out of them so you might have the ability to release the stress of these loops that can keep you from letting go into sleep.

Mindfulness Exercise #1: Ready. Set. DO NOTHING.

I have a one minute mindfulness exercise I teach as one of the main ways for tackling the going stress that is a major contributor to insomnia. If you want to reliably get to sleep and sleep deeply it is critical to learn to stop and do nothing because that's basically what you're doing when you sleep. Yes, your brain and body are very busy recovering while you sleep, but you are doing nothing. When you stop and do nothing during the day, even if it's only for one minute, your brain and body learn to shift from going and doing to stillness and rest. The more you do this, the more op-portunities your brain and body have to learn that life has a rhythm, an alternating rhythm of going and stillness, of doing and resting.

Here's the "1-Minute DO Nothing" exercise:

You can do this anytime, but it's best to connect it to something you do several times per day. I use it just before I start my car and just before I get out of the car. That way I will do it at least four times per day.

1. Stop

2. Set a timer for one minute

3. Make sure to follow step two; it's what keeps us honest (we are all natural cheaters when it comes to doing nothing)

4. With eyes open, take in sights and sounds, simply observing the whole experience of your surroundings

5. If you care to, close your eyes and check-in on the condition of your mind and body

6. As you do steps 4 and 5, notice any urge to go and then just keep doing nothing

7. When your minute is up simply go on with your day

When you first start doing this exercise, it will probably feel awkward at best and like finger nails on a chalk board (do those even exist anymore?) at worst. That's OK. That's how you're supposed to feel when you interrupt the flow of going and doing with something as bizarre as actually pausing to do nothing. As you become an expert at doing nothing, any feelings of discomfort will probably pass. Daily mindfulness practice is important and every practice counts as a success, even if it's only a minute.

Mindfulness Exercise #2:
"I am _____ and I know that I am _____."

Here is a technique for changing your experience of tangles. One way to increase mindfulness is to bring attention to exactly what you are doing at any given moment. This is a technique I like to use to untangle myself from work when I get home at the end of each day. I do it while I'm changing into more comfortable clothes (believe it or not I don't always wear stuffy business shirts), but you can use it wherever it fits for you (maybe getting ready for bed?).

- As you take off each piece of clothing say to yourself, "As I remove this _____ (sock, shirt, etc...), I set aside my work/responsibilities/worries until tomorrow."

- As you put on each piece of your pajamas or take each step in your bedtime routine say to yourself, "As I _____, I invite my mind and body to rest and recover fully and completely."

- You might end up saying each of these phrases to yourself 5-10 times in the process of changing clothes or going through your evening routine. This repetition serves to refocus your mind away from tangles and in the direction of rest and recovery.

The more general version of this exercise, which you can use anytime you want to be more mindful, is to repeat in your mind the phrase, "I am _____ and I know that I am _____." An example might be, "I am walking and I know that I am walking." Or, "I am eating and I know that I am eating." Or, "I am driving and I know that I am driving."

Conclusion

This chapter started with the words, "If you're not stressed you're dead." I believe that unless you have a regular meditation, relaxation, or prayer practice focused on changing the way you relate to stress, then stress is almost certainly a source of insomnia. It can also be a source of vulnerability for relapse into another episode of insomnia once you get better. For this reason, I also encourage everyone to cultivate a long-term daily practice. With daily practice you will develop a high degree of skill that will serve you when you really need it.

PART 4

PERSONAL SLEEP TRANSFORMATION
AND THE INSOMNIA CLINIC™

CHAPTER 14

PERSONAL SLEEP TRANSFORMATION: HOW TO OBEY THE LAW

If you've made it this far then you've read at least 10 chapters, you know the 10 Laws of Insomnia, and you know there are simple yet challenging ways to take control of insomnia and reclaim your best life. This chapter summarizes all of the strategies from the last 10 chapters into one place so you can begin to craft a personal sleep transformation plan. Applying these strategies can be challenging so there's also an exercise for creating a compelling vision of your best life without insomnia, a vision that motivates you to make the changes that will make it a reality.

The Rest of Your Insomnia Story:

You wrote the beginning of your sleep story in chapter 4 (LAW #1: Sleep is Critically Essential). If you didn't, I encourage you to take a few minutes to do it now. Taking an honest look at how your sleep problem is affecting your life helps to clarify why you are here and give you the motivation to take action to change your sleep. However, understanding and awareness of how insomnia is affecting you, your health, your life, and your relationships is not enough to keep you committed and motivated through the process of sleep transformation. You also need a compelling vision of what you're working toward. You need a compelling vision of your best life without insomnia.

Use the questions and space below to write the ending of your sleep story. What will your life be like after you have mastered insomnia? I want you to be specific. Why do you care about sleeping better? What's going to change when you do? I want you to give it some real thought. After all, this is your life we're talking about.

Everyone says things like, "I'll have more energy" and "I won't be so grouchy." These are true. Who doesn't want to be more energetic and less moody? But they aren't very motivating, they're not exciting, and they are definitely not compelling. What is exciting is how your life will be different when you are more energetic and in a better mood. Why do you want to be in a better mood? What would you be doing with more energy if you had it and how would those things make your life better? These are the things I would be excited to read about in your sleep story.

Take a few minutes now to write the ending of your sleep story:

1. What will you DO differently on a day-to-day basis when you're sleeping well? Finish this sentence: When I wake up well rested every day I will... (e.g. hike, say yes to friends, play with the kids, clean the house, etc...)

   _____

   _____

   _____

2. How would you describe yourself when you're well rested? WHO are you as a parent, friend, partner, boss, student, or employee when you're sleeping great? Finish this sentence: When I'm sleeping great I am...

   _____

   _____

   _____

3. List the ways you're better when getting <u>plenty of restful sleep</u> on a regular basis (e.g. more energetic, mentally sharp, more patient, better mood, etc...):

_____

_____

_____

_____

_____

_____

_____

_____

4. When you're better in all of the ways listed in question three, how will you be different with your spouse, children, parents, and siblings? How will relationships with family members be better?

_____

_____

_____

_____

_____

_____

5. When you're better in all of the ways listed in question three, how will you be different with friends? How will friendships be better?

_____

_____

_____

_____

_____

_____

_____

_____

6. When you're better in all of the ways listed in question three, how will you be different at work? How will your performance, satisfaction, and relationships at work be better?

_____

_____

_____

_____

_____

_____

_____

7. When you're better in all of the ways listed in question three, how will your health change? How will your physical, emotional, and psycho-logical health improve?

_____

_____

_____

_____

_____

_____

Hold on to this. Put it where you can see it often. When you get to the challenging parts of the sleep transformation program, this part of your sleep story will remind you why it's all worthwhile.

Summary of the 10 Laws of Insomnia and Sleep Transformation Strategies

The life you describe above is possible, even likely. You now have the tools to start taking control of insomnia and creating your best life now. It's time to create a sleep transformation plan. Here is a summary of the laws and strategies you've learned throughout the book. Review them in preparation for creating your plan.

Law #1: Sleep is Critically Essential

Exercise: What's your sleep story?

The sleep story exercise is about motivation. It helps you clarify how insomnia drags down your life, health, and relationships. This is important because the pain and discomfort of any problem is a large part of what motivates us to make the changes necessary to solve the problem.

Law #2: Insomnia Has Many Causes

Exercise: Basic Sleep Discovery - Solving the Puzzle

The basic sleep discovery exercise is about understanding the sources of your insomnia. When you look at your insomnia through the lens of this exercise you will begin to have a "big picture" perspective. This exercise will also help you identify clear reasons for insomnia that support you in taking specific actions toward getting better.

Law #3: Insomnia Has a Life of Its' Own

Exercise: No Excuses - Read Chapter Again

The exercise for this law is to read the chapter again for the purpose of building even more understanding and motivation. The information in this chapter lays the foundation for why it is almost certainly possible for you to take control of insomnia without pills regardless of age or any other health problems you may have.

Law #4: Insomnia is a Tricky Problem
Exercise: Five Success Obstacles - Read Chapter Again

The exercise for this chapter is also to read the chapter again. Again, the purpose is to build even more understanding and motivation. The information in this chapter will protect you from the thoughts, beliefs, and approaches to insomnia that lead to unnecessary failure. If you are familiar with these obstacles it will be much easier to overcome them when they arise during your sleep transformation process.

Law #5: Insomnia is a Power Problem
Exercise: Four Power Boosts

The four power boosts are the beginning of the rapid insomnia relief strategies. Your sleep power controls your readiness for sleep and the depth and quality of your sleep and you have control over sleep power. By choosing when you will go to bed, when you will get up, how much time you spend in bed, and how you use naps, you have the ability to actively manipulate your sleep power.

Law #6: Insomnia is a Programming Problem
Exercise: Reprogram - Escape. Hang Out. Try Again.

Escape, Hang Out, Try Again is the second half of the rapid insomnia relief strategy. Combined with the four power boosts, consistently responding to your experience of sleeplessness with this strategy will likely get you a meaningful improvement in your sleep pattern in 2-3 weeks, maybe in just a few days.

Law #7: Insomnia is a Mind Problem
Exercise: Thinking - Identify. Challenge. Rethink.

Identify, Challenge, and Rethink is the first of the advanced insomnia relief techniques. If you struggle with general worries or worries about sleep that cause mental or physical activation and sleeplessness, then this should definitely be a part of your sleep transformation plan. Your mind can be a powerful force that leads you towards or away from blissful sleep.

Law #8: Sleep is Slippery
Exercise: Playing Hard to Get

This exercise is about escaping the trap of trying too hard to get to sleep. If you find yourself spending significant time and effort figuring out how you can get sleep then this will be an important part of your plan. Amazing things happen when you give up on the desperate pursuit of sleep.

Law #9: Insomnia is a 24-Hour Problem
Exercise: 24-Hour Activity and Experience Tracking

This exercise is about expanding your perspective on where the sources and solutions for insomnia can be found. If your insomnia seems to be coming out of the blue with no clear cause then you will likely find it useful to include 24-hour activity and experience tracking in your plan.

Law #10: Insomnia is a Stress Problem
Exercise: Mindfulness Training

Stress is universal but we all handle it differently. Do you find that worry, tension, over activation, and a sense of overwhelm are a routine part of your day-to-day experience? If so, then stress is likely a part of your insomnia puzzle. Stress management techniques take weeks of daily practice to be fully effective so start them early in the process if you think stress is a major player for you. Regardless of your level of stress, a daily meditation practice has broad benefits for health and quality of life. Because of this, I encourage everyone in the sleep transformation program to develop a daily practice.

Personalized Sleep Transformation Plan

One approach to sleep transformation using this book is to look at the summary above and focus your efforts on the exercises and strategies that resonate most strongly with you. From this you will craft a plan that contains the sleep transformation strategies you believe are the most relevant and most likely to lead to meaningful change in your sleep and your life. If you're a lone wolf and you do best doing things your own way, then this may be the most effective way to go about your personal sleep transformation. However, for most people (even some lone wolves) the recommended plan below will be more effective.

Recommended Sleep Transformation Plan

I have written this book with the chapters, laws, and exercises in the order I believe is likely to be most beneficial for you. With this in mind I've outlined four basic steps for using the information in the book. Before I outline these steps, however, I'd like to share some general suggestions about how to handle sleep medications while you're in the sleep transformation process.

Thoughts about Sleep Medication during Sleep Transformation Training

As with any health related issue, you should always consult with and follow the direction of your healthcare provider. This includes any decision to start, stop, or change your use of sleep medications. As far as starting medications, I understand that sleep is important and sometimes the only way to meet an urgent need for sleep is to take a pill. With that said, if you're not taking sleep medication now then my suggestion is that you don't start. After a few weeks of sleep transformation training it is likely that you will be sleeping fine without the help of a pill.

When it comes to stopping or changing your use of sleep medications, the situation is a bit trickier. You can read the chapter on sleep medications later in the book to understand what I mean by this but for now just know that it can be tricky. I have two general suggestions:

1. If you're sleeping well with your medication but would like to stop taking it, then you will likely need to begin reducing the dose of the medication at the same time or shortly after you start the rapid insomnia relief strategies. If you're in this situation, please speak with your healthcare provider to get guidance before making any change in your sleep medication.

2. If you are sleeping poorly with your sleep medications, then I suggest that you just keep taking it as you have been for the time being. My thinking on this is that it's useful to strengthen your natural sleep systems and get you sleeping better before "pulling the rug out from under you" by trying to reduce sleep medications. I find that people are able to approach the process of reducing or eliminating sleep medication with much more confidence and success when they are sleeping well and are well rested.

Four Steps to Using the Information and Strategies in This Book

1. Read and complete the exercises in Chapters 4 and 5 to fully understand your insomnia, its effect on your life, and the targets for your sleep transformation.

2. Read Chapters 6 and 7 to build belief in the possibility that you can get better and to gain confidence that you know how to approach the sleep transformation process.

3. Read Chapters 8 and 9 thoroughly and commit to a 21 day period that you will follow the rapid insomnia relief strategies consistently and to the best of your ability. During this time you can read the chapters on advanced insomnia relief but I want your energy focused only on the rapid relief strategies for the first 21 days.

4. After 21 days of following the rapid relief strategies, you should be experiencing a significant improvement in your sleep pattern. Continue using these strategies as needed and start implementing the advanced insomnia relief strategies in Chapters 10-13. I suggest adding only one strategy every 1-2 weeks. This will give you time to get familiar with and develop a basic level of skill with each strategy.

Final Thoughts

If you follow this plan there is a good chance you will experience radically improved sleep and life satisfaction in just a few weeks. If this is the case I want to hear all about it. Especially the part about how taking control of insomnia has begun to catapult you into living your best life.

However, if you're not experiencing radically better sleep after 4-6 weeks of following this plan then it's time to contact The Insomnia Clinic or a healthcare provider. You're probably going to need some help. The next couple of chapters will help you get familiar with how The Insomnia Clinic works and what to expect if you decide you need help taking control of insomnia.

CHAPTER 15

THE INSOMNIA CLINIC PART I: SOLVING THE PUZZLE WITH GUIDED SLEEP DISCOVERY™

At The Insomnia Clinic we have a system called Guided Sleep Discovery for helping you solve your puzzle of poor sleep. Your sleep discovery will follow a three step process of identifying the causes of poor sleep, prioritizing their importance, and creating a plan to systematically address them.

Guided Sleep Discovery

Guided Sleep Discovery is a process of learning exactly what is causing your experience of insomnia. Together with your insomnia specialist, you will examine these 12 sources of insomnia.

- Insomnia and Sleeplessness
- Sleepiness and Fatigue
- Circadian Rhythms (Body Clock)
- Movements and Sleep
- Sleep Apnea
- Health and Illness
- Stress
- Happiness
- Lifestyle
- Sleep Medication
- Caffeine, Alcohol, and Other Stuff
- Nightmares, Sleepwalking, and Unusual Stuff

This is not a generic process. Your sleep discovery will involve identifying all of the factors that are causing or worsening your insomnia and carefully determining the degree that each of these is actually driving your insomnia. This process can often be completed during the first discovery session with your insomnia specialist. However, it may also include follow-up meetings for specialized testing, extended sleep tracking or overnight sleep studies. These advanced sleep discovery technologies are described in more detail at the end of this chapter.

Once your specific insomnia factors are identified, you will work closely with your insomnia specialist to create a plan with specific recommendations for addressing each factor. This will likely include Radical Sleep Transformation, but may also include assessment and/or treatment for other sleep disorders and coordination with your other healthcare providers.

Summary of the 12 Sources of Insomnia

Insomnia and Sleeplessness

Trouble getting to sleep or staying asleep? Plenty of sleep, but never feel rested? Insomnia comes in many shapes and sizes. Determining the "shape" of your sleep (or lack of it) is the first step of the sleep discovery process.

Sleepiness and Fatigue

When do you feel at your best? When do you feel at your worst? Are you sleepy or just tired? There's a difference and it's important. How you feel while awake provides critical information about your sleep problem and how to move you from surviving to thriving.

Circadian Rhythms (Body Clock)

Ever feel like your days and nights are mixed up? A powerful internal clock controls when your body and brain want to be awake and asleep. Understanding and solving your sleep problem requires knowing how your internal clock is set and what kind of clock you have.

Health and Illness

Headaches, arthritis, depression, cancer, anxiety, tinnitus, Parkinson's disease, and many other health problems interfere with sleep, but illness does not equal insomnia. Are you a hopeless case or can you sleep and feel better despite these problems? Guided Sleep Discovery will help you find the answer.

Stress

Good stress. Bad Stress. We all have it. The trick is to know how it influences you and when to do something about it. Guided Sleep Discovery includes a powerful stress check to understand your stress and how it may be leaking out in your sleep.

Sleep Apnea

What do you know about sleep apnea? It only happens in overweight men who snore? Not quite. If you have stubborn insomnia you may have silent sleep apnea. Guided Sleep Discovery looks deeply to learn if sleep apnea may be a problem for you.

Caffeine, Alcohol, and Other Stuff

Good, bad, or ugly, anything that affects your brain affects your sleep. What's the latest you should drink caffeine? Does alcohol help or just make insomnia worse? What about other drugs like marijuana? Your habits can lead to blissful nights and vibrant days...or not.

Happiness

Some of the most stubborn insomnia problems are happiness problems. Whether it is work, finances, health, family, or relationships, dissatisfaction has a funny way of disrupting sleep. Guided Sleep Discovery uses sophisticated tools for understanding your degree of life satisfaction, its potential effect on your sleep, and its role as a support or obstacle in your personal sleep transformation.

Lifestyle

Great sleep is essential for living your best life, but how does your life impact your sleep? For better or worse, the things we do while awake influence the level of bliss and restoration we experience during sleep. Do you act like a good sleeper? Guided Sleep Discovery will let you know.

Sleep Medication

Sleeping pills can be a blessing and a curse. They can be a lifesaver in the short term but over time they may be a barrier to deep sleep. Nobody wants to be dependent on a pill, especially when it's not working. Are you addicted? Can you get free of them? Is that even a good idea? Guided Sleep Discovery will help you find the answers.

Movements and Sleep

Do your legs keep you awake? What are they doing while you're sleeping? Do you really want to know? Sleep discovery reveals key signs of Restless Legs Syndrome and "wiggles" that may keep you from ever feeling rested.

Nightmares, Sleepwalking, and Unusual Stuff

Some things that happen during sleep can be dangerous, mysterious and frightening. When you know how sleep works they usually make sense. Guided Sleep Discovery uncovers why they're happening and how to get rid of them.

The Sleep Discovery Interview

Your first meeting at The Insomnia Clinic will last 20 to 90 minutes and involves a lot of questions and quite a bit of paperwork. Together with your insomnia specialist you will begin to look closely at the 12 Sources of Insomnia in search of anything and everything that may be negatively affecting your sleep. You will then perform a careful analysis of all factors you have identified and work to come up with a prioritized "map" of...

1. Specific factors causing your insomnia

2. The contribution of each factor to the problem

3. Exactly how to address each factor through a targeted program of further evaluation and Radical Sleep Transformation

What to Expect From Your Insomnia Specialist

If you were able to overcome your insomnia on your own, you would not be looking to The Insomnia Clinic as a resource. However, you are an expert on your own body. You are also an expert on your history and experience of insomnia. This is a central understanding from which we operate at The Insomnia Clinic. We've learned that your personal expertise, combined with our knowledge and experience, make a powerful formula for success. This means that the relationship you have with your insomnia specialist is one of collaboration. From this foundation of collaboration, your insomnia specialist will support and build you up in several ways to help you overcome any challenges or obstacles standing in the way of your radical sleep transformation.

Expert training

You will receive a mix of the most proven and the most cutting edge methods for sleep transformation, some of which were created by and available only through The Insomnia Clinic.

Hope

We know there's a solution to every sleep problem. Beginning with your discovery session, you'll receive a concrete plan for achieving your best sleep and your best life through sleep transformation.

Clarity

You've probably noticed that everyone seems to have advice. "Try this, it worked for me." "Try that, my mother-in-law loves it." We'll show you clear and workable strategies for taking control of insomnia.

Unique Path

You're not like everyone else. The "cookie cutter" plan doesn't work for you. You'll receive a plan and strategies that make up a tailored sleep solution unique to your specific puzzle of poor sleep.

Accountability and Confidence

Even when you know what you need to do, making sleep health changes on your own can be daunting. We'll be right beside you along the way, so you can make each step of sleep transformation with confidence. We'll hold you accountable, so you can follow through when it's tough.

Support

We'll be your cheerleader and advisor. When you have questions, we'll have answers.

Advanced Sleep Discovery Technology

Your sleep transformation plan may include using professional hi-tech assessment tools to help us uncover the mystery of your insomnia. Technologies frequently used at The Insomnia Clinic include extended sleep tracking, overnight sleep studies, and psychological testing.

Overnight Sleep Studies

Just because you have a sleep problem does not mean you need a sleep study. However, a sleep study (which can now be done at home or in a sleep laboratory) can tell us exactly what your brain and body are doing during the night and remains the only way to accurately learn if breathing or movement problems during the night are a major cause of your sleep problem. Do you think you don't have a breathing problem? Think again.

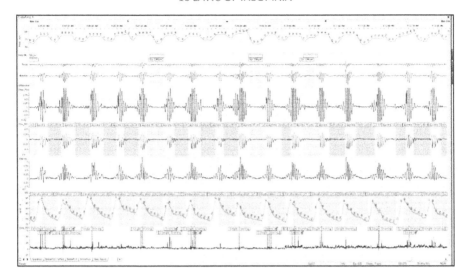

Figure 1. Sleep Study Recording

Many healthcare providers recommend sleep studies simply because they don't understand the sleep problem well enough and think it's "just the next thing to do." In The Insomnia Clinic, during your sleep discovery interview we help you make the decision about whether or not the stress and cost of a sleep study is necessary, based on the fullest understanding of your insomnia puzzle. If you've already had a sleep study, we will help you understand what it says, what it means, and what you should do about it.

Psychological Testing

When a sleep problem becomes stubborn or complicated, advanced information that provides sophisticated understanding of thinking, feeling, and problem solving patterns helps us to come to a deep understanding of the sleep problem itself. This information also guides us to the strategies for fixing your sleep problem that are likely to be most successful for you. At The Insomnia Clinic we use some of the most advanced and well researched testing available to help us identify:

- Personality patterns that help (or hinder) the process of improving sleep

- Thinking patterns that fuel the fires of stress and sleeplessness

- Emotional patterns that cause fatigue and promote illness

- Behavior patterns that drain sleep power

Extended Sleep Tracking (Wrist Actigraphy Assessment)

Are you getting more sleep than you realize? Dozing off in the evenings without even knowing it? Do you think your sleep schedule is turned upside down? Sleepy all the time? Tried "everything" to fix your sleep problem but nothing seems to work? It may be time to take a closer look at your sleep patterns and find out what's really happening at night.

An actigraph is one of the most powerful and advanced ways to measure your sleep and wake patterns in a way no other technology can. It's more powerful than the sleep watch you got off the internet and way more advanced than the free app you downloaded onto your smartphone. By measuring light and movement every minute of every hour of every day for up to 15 days, this tiny piece of big technology provides a close-up view of your sleep pattern. In fact, it can measure sleep with up to 90% accuracy.

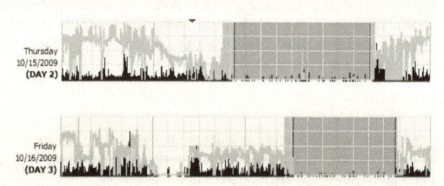

Figure 2. 48-Hour "Snapshot" of Actigraphy Assessment

Actigraphy assessment is often a critical part of the diagnosis and treatment of insomnia, circadian rhythm (body clock) problems, excessive sleepiness, and other sleep disorders. In collaboration with your insomnia specialist, information from this technology may be the key to helping you and your provider:

- Understand exactly what type of insomnia you have

- Choose the correct treatment for your insomnia

- Identify and understand factors causing your insomnia or keeping you from getting better

How is actigraphy different than a sleep study?

Where an overnight sleep study evaluates sleep breathing and movement problems during a single night, an actigraph records your 24-hour sleep-wake patterns for up to 15 days while you go about your normal day-to-day routines.

We've made the Discovery. Now What?

This sleep discovery process is powerful. In fact, many of the folks who come to The Insomnia Clinic are pleasantly surprised at how quickly we can develop a deep and clear understanding about an insomnia problem that has seemed to remain a stubborn mystery, despite many previous efforts. With a clear understanding and a plan, it's time to get to work on Radical Sleep Transformation.

CHAPTER 16

THE INSOMNIA CLINIC PART II: GETTING TO WORK ON RADICAL SLEEP TRANSFORMATION™

Once you've completed the sleep discovery process and crafted your personalized sleep transformation plan, it's time to get to work on Radical Sleep Transformation.

Radical Sleep Transformation

During your sleep transformation program, you will meet regularly with an insomnia specialist who personally guides you through the scientifically proven process of reversing brain changes caused by insomnia, strengthening your natural sleep system, and removing obstacles to great sleep. Your insomnia specialist will provide clear instruction on how to start each aspect of your plan. You will then follow-up with your insomnia specialist on a regular basis to monitor successes, identify obstacles, and continuously modify and adjust your plan until you're sleeping better.

The Radical Sleep Transformation program is designed to teach you the information and strategies you need to create restful satisfying sleep that energizes you for your best life. While in the sleep transformation program, you will work with an insomnia specialist to leverage the 10 Sources of Sleep Transformation.

10 Sources of Sleep Transformation

RAPID INSOMNIA RELIEF STRATEGIES

We want you sleeping better fast. You will immediately learn the simple and powerful changes in sleep behavior that are proven to quickly break down insomnia and boost the power of your natural sleep systems. These strategies are designed and proven to change the way your brain structures sleep, so you can start falling asleep faster, wake up less, experience better quality sleep, and simply get more sleep in as little as 14 days.

BREAKING DOWN BARRIERS

What's standing between you and a refreshing night of sleep? We'll help you take effective action to eliminate any barriers to sleep that are identified during your sleep discovery process. Whether it's chronic pain, depression, sleep apnea, or another illness or a sleep disorder, we'll provide recommendations and connections for breaking down these barriers.

UNDERSTANDING SLEEP AND INSOMNIA

Learn the secrets of sleep and the brain that give you the power to control insomnia. When you know how sleep and insomnia systems work, you can create the highly satisfying sleep pattern you need and desire.

THE RIDICULOUS ART OF DOING NOTHING

Sleep is tricky. The harder you try, the harder it is. Learn advanced methods for bringing stillness to the mind and body so your natural sleep systems can effortlessly take over. You will use these methods to master stress, making your natural sleep more resilient and impervious to stress.

ENHANCED RECOVERY DEMAND

Although scientists have yet to fully understand the exact purpose of sleep, we do know it is essential for recovery and restoration of the body and brain. We'll focus on teaching you to use your mind and body throughout the day in a way that generates maximum need for peaceful restorative sleep.

THE TEFLON MIND OF THE GREAT SLEEPER

A restless mind is the enemy of peaceful nights. Learn powerful strategies for controlling a stubborn mind. Uncover the thoughts and beliefs about sleep that fuel insomnia and replace them with those of a great sleeper.

HEALTHY SLEEP HABITS

These are the everyday things that give you the best chance for a good night's sleep. When should you exercise? What's the latest you should drink caffeine? What about dinner? Do you have to eliminate every ray of light from your bedroom? What about smartphones and tablets, will the light from the screens keep you awake? Although keeping healthy habits won't fix insomnia, it will support your sleep transformation efforts.

DROPS OF JOY: GROWING HAPPINESS

Small changes, done every day, make for big growth toward maximum happiness. We'll teach you a set of techniques for building joy and satisfaction in relationships, at work, in your mind, and in your body. We believe that increased life satisfaction equals increased sleep satisfaction and our goal is to help you boost them both.

SLEEPING PILL ESCAPE PLAN

In collaboration with your prescriber, we'll help you come up with a plan for stopping sleep medication safely, while maintaining a healthy satisfying sleep pattern. You may not want or need to stop taking sleep medication, but you probably can if you choose to. The reality is that you may actually sleep better once you stop them. There is nothing like natural sleep.

INSOMNIA PREVENTION TRAINING

Once you've created a highly satisfying sleep pattern, the program will turn toward ensuring you know the causes of your insomnia and, more importantly, exactly what you did to fix it. With this knowledge you will create a plan for how to maintain optimal sleep long-term in the face of future challenges life will inevitably present.

Commitment to Sleep Transformation

On average, the process of sleep transformation involves 6-8 visits with an insomnia specialist over a period of 6-12 weeks. Although basic insomnia relief usually takes only 2-6 weeks, full recovery from insomnia and installing of the empowering factors that truly maximize sleep satisfaction and minimize risk for future insomnia take a bit longer. A typical appointment is between 20 and 40 minutes long. Your individual sleep transformation could be shorter or longer, depending of the nature of your sleep puzzle. For example, insomnia combined with anxiety or depression usually takes somewhat longer to transform. Also, if you've been taking sleeping pills for more than a couple of months, it may take us a few extra visits to help you achieve a high degree of sleep satisfaction free from pills. On the other hand, if you're generally healthy and highly motivated to take effective action, we may be able to transform your insomnia in just a few weeks.

Time to Get to Work

Regardless of your situation, it's important to remember there is a solution to every sleep problem, and the sleep transformation program provides a clear path to your best sleep and your best life. If our systematic approach to insomnia makes sense to you then don't wait any longer. Contact The Insomnia Clinic to schedule your Guided Sleep Discovery session and start down the path toward your personal sleep transformation.

PART 5

BEYOND THE LAWS OF INSOMNIA

CHAPTER 17

THE TRUTH ABOUT SLEEP MEDICATION

From what you've read so far, you may have the impression that I have a fanatical dislike for sleep medications. Let me take a moment to make my opinions about sleep medications clear. Sleep medications like Ambien, Lunesta, and others have a critical role in our healthcare system. They help millions of Americans sleep better and, through better sleep, live healthier happier lives. The most obvious appropriate use of sleep medications is for insomnia that occurs as a result of short-term stress or illness. Another is chronic illness that directly interferes with sleep and the insomnia caused by the illness cannot be eliminated in any other way. Regardless of the situation, if the choice is between not sleeping and using a sleep medication, then I will almost always encourage use of the medication. The consequences of insomnia are too significant to go on unmanaged.

With that said, in my opinion, long term use of sleep medication (more than a few weeks) is risky and unnecessary in most cases. In the remainder of this chapter I will share with you the information and experience that led me to hold this opinion. The short version can be summarized in three points:

- All sleep medications carry a risk for addiction and other potentially dangerous effects.

- Sleep transformation training, like that taught in this book, is as effective as any sleep medication.

- Most people can achieve a satisfactory sleep pattern without medication.

What Medications Am I Talking About?

I'm not going to get into the details of all of the medications used for sleep. There's just not enough space in this book to do that. Just understand that although there are many similarities, each medication used for insomnia is a little bit different in terms of how it affects sleep, potential side effects, and risk for physical or psychological dependence. Here is a list of common medications used for treating insomnia:

Ambien (zolpidem)	Prosom (estazolam)	Desyrel (trazodone)
Ambien CR (zolpidem)	Dalmane (flurazepam)	Elavil (amitriptyline)
Intermezzo (zolpidem)	Doral (quazepam)	Seroquel (quetiapine)
Lunesta (eszopiclone)	Restoril (temazepam)	Remeron (mirtazapine)
Sonata (zaleplon)	Halcion (triazolam)	Surmontil (trimipramine)
Rozerem (ramelteon)	Ativan (lorazepam)	Zyprexa (olanzapine)
Silenor (doxepin)	Xanax (alprazolam)	
Belsomra (suvorexant)	Klonopin (clonazepam)	

Traditional Healthcare Approach to Insomnia

To talk about the first point - risk of addiction and other dangerous effects - I'll describe the most common "pathways" or experiences you might have when trying to address your insomnia within our healthcare system. The way the traditional healthcare system deals with insomnia is fairly predictable. The almost universal approach is to prescribe a medication and provide a handout of healthy sleep tips. Because of this, people with insomnia often wait years before talking to their healthcare provider about insomnia because they don't really want a medication to help them sleep.

When the conversation about insomnia is started, whether by the insomnia sufferer or by the healthcare provider, the evaluation of the sleep problem may range anywhere from a few questions about sleep patterns to a deeper conversation about sleep, health, and factors influencing insomnia. The process may also involve additional diagnostic tests. However, the research tells us that most sleep problems in primary care go undiagnosed and untreated. One reason for this is that providers have extremely limited time to speak with patients about many health concerns.

As I've said before, sleep medications play an important and essential role in the care for insomnia. However, almost all of these medications were intended to be used for normal and short episodes of insomnia that happen in the face of normal life stressors and go away after a few weeks. In fact, the FDA recommendation for most sleep drugs is that they should be taken for no more than 14 days. Unfortunately, this rarely happens. Once started on a sleep medication, the average person ends up taking them for at least a year; sometimes for decades. There are five main "pathways" you are likely to experience if you decide to use sleep medication.

Pathway #1: Unhappy Refuser

You might try a sleep medication but find yourself unhappy for some reason and ultimately decide to stop using it. This may be because you are simply uncomfortable with the possible short and long-term effects and risks of the medication. Or because you experienced intolerable or dangerous effects such as excessive daytime sleepiness or dangerous behaviors during sleep (e.g. eating, driving, or sexual activity) while using sleep medication. Whatever the reason, you decide that any benefit of the medication doesn't warrant the risks.

Pathway #2: Happy Occasional User

Most prescriptions for sleep medication start with a recommendation to use them as needed a few nights per week or a few nights per month. You may be satisfied using a sleep medication in this way. You take a sleeping pill when you're feeling a bit worn down from a couple of bad nights' sleep. Or maybe you take one when you need to be sure of good night's sleep before a big day. Use of a sleep medication in this way prevents you from experiencing any significant consequences of insomnia and can prevent some of the mind problems discussed in Chapter 10 (Law #8: Insomnia is a Mind Problem). You might go on using sleep medication in this fashion for many years with no problems at all. However, as many people do, you may over time find yourself using sleep medication more and more often. This can lead to dependence on the medication and entry into pathways three, four, or five.

Pathway #3: Happy and Dependent

For the most part, if you are in this pathway you experience elimination of your insomnia symptoms, get satisfying restful sleep most nights, and feel rested and energetic during the daytime. You have no significant side effects associated with use of sleep medication and you're comfortable taking the medication on a long-term basis. This sounds okay, right? There are two problems you might experience. First, you may become trapped. What do I mean by trapped? You're trapped when you become dependent on the medication to sleep and any attempt to reduce or eliminate the medication causes a return of insomnia symptoms and sometimes a worsening of insomnia symptoms called "rebound insomnia." Rebound Insomnia is a situation in which the insomnia experienced when trying to stop a sleep medication is more severe than the insomnia the medication was used to treat. Second, over time your sleep medication may become less effective or fail to work altogether. Due to this second problem, you may ultimately find yourself in pathway number four, unhappy and dependent.

Pathway #4: Unhappy and Dependent

If you're in this pathway, your sleep medication is helping, but only partially. You're definitely sleeping better with medication than without it. However, you continue to have significant problems with nighttime sleep or daytime dissatisfaction despite using sleep medication. After a matter of time your body develops a dependence on the medication and you will probably experience rebound insomnia if you try to reduce or stop using the medication.

You may also find yourself in this pathway after spending some time in pathway number three, happy and dependent. Whether it was a period of months or maybe even years, you experienced great satisfaction with use of sleep medication. However, for some reason your sleep medication no longer works as well as it once did or has stopped working altogether. You're no longer satisfied with your sleep or daytime experience. Attempts to reduce or stop the medication result in a return of insomnia symptoms. You're no longer satisfied with the benefits of the medication but are unable to stop taking it. There is also a possibility that you are experiencing some kind of unwanted effects from the medication, and continuing to pay for it month after month despite the fact that it's not working.

If you're in this pathway you've most likely experienced a cycle of repeated recommendations from your healthcare provider to increase the dose of your sleep medication, switch to another medication, or add an additional medication. If sleep medications are not working well for you, sooner or later your provider will probably develop a suspicion that they are not working because your insomnia is caused by anxiety or depression. Most commonly, this will lead him or her to recommend some kind of antidepressant medication. In some unfortunate situations, this unhappy and dependent pathway turns into the final pathway - unhappy, dependent and hung out to dry.

Pathway #5: Unhappy, Dependent, and Hung Out to Dry

If you are in this pathway, you are working with a healthcare provider who is uncomfortable prescribing your sleep medication. This can happen for many (usually very good) reasons. Your prescriber may feel that continued use of sleep medication is unsafe or inappropriate because of a change in your health status, changes in other medications, new information about the sleep medication, or development of dangerous side effects. You may also come across healthcare providers who believe that sleep medications are generally unsafe or inappropriate and refuse to prescribe them. You may experience this when changing to a new healthcare provider. Obviously, it is problematic when you have become dependent on sleep medication and your prescriber has determined (usually for good reasons) that it is unsafe or inappropriate for you to continue to use it.

There is usually an effort to taper off of the medication. However, these efforts are often unsuccessful, leaving individuals with intolerable insomnia symptoms and no treatment options. Individuals in this situation frequently come to The Insomnia Clinic feeling desperate in the face of stubborn insomnia symptoms and feeling they have nowhere to turn. In the best cases, healthcare providers will refer folks to The Insomnia Clinic to initiate non-medication treatment and slow reductions of sleep medication over time.

Final Thoughts on the Traditional Insomnia Pathways

If you look at these five pathways, you will see that the traditional strategy for managing insomnia within our healthcare system isn't working. Four of the five pathways lead to one of two outcomes.

- Refuse medication and continue to suffer with insomnia

- Become dependent on sleep medication and hope for the best

Sadly, many providers and insomnia sufferers feel these are the only two options. Fortunately this is untrue. The remainder of this chapter will show you why.

Sleep Transformation Training versus Sleep Medication

Sleep medication is the most frequently recommended therapy for managing insomnia.[1] This is despite the fact that there is no research evidence to support a preference for sleep medication over cognitive-behavioral treatment.[2] In fact, there is more research on cognitive-behavioral treatment for insomnia (What I call Radical Sleep Transformation or sleep transformation training) than on any single sleep medication available. The research says that sleep transformation training is effective if you have simple insomnia.[3] It is also effective if you have more complicated insomnia that is present along with other health problems.[4-13] See Chapter 6 (LAW #3: Insomnia Has a Life of Its Own) for a discussion of what scientific research says about sleep transformation training for various types of insomnia. **Basically, this research clearly shows that sleep transformation training is an effective option for managing insomnia all by itself.**

There have been some great research studies published that directly compare the effects of medication to those of sleep transformation training. I'll tell you about two of them here. The Journal of the American Medical Association (JAMA) published one of the most rigorous clinical trials comparing sleep transformation training to the sleep drug Ambien in 2009.[3] In this study, 90% of insomnia patients experienced clinically significant improvement and 40% experienced complete remission of insomnia symptoms. Sleep transformation training was as effective as medication, and whereas long-term medication use led to an increase in insomnia symptoms, participants who used sleep transformation training continued to experience growing improvements in their sleep up to a year after they stopped the treatment. Why is this? While sleep medications mask or cover up insomnia symptoms, sleep transformation training changes many of the actual causes responsible for chronic insomnia.

Another study compared the effectiveness of sleep transformation and medication by analyzing the data from 21 different studies using a powerful mathematical process called meta-analysis.[14] The researchers found that both medication and sleep transformation training each led to moderate to large improvements in the ability to fall asleep, the ability to stay asleep, and the amount of time spent awake during the night. In fact, the improvements in sleep achieved by each method were nearly identical, with one exception. Sleep transformation training was significantly better than medication at helping people fall asleep faster. **These two studies tell us that sleep transformation training leads to improvements in sleep equal to or better than those from medications and the benefits from sleep transformation training last well after you're done with training.**

Not only are the improvements from sleep transformation training as good or better than those from medication, but there is some question as to whether the sleep inducing chemicals in newer medications are actually responsible for the improvements in sleep. Another meta-analysis published in 2012 analyzed 13 studies comparing sleep medications to placebo in more than 4000 people with insomnia.[15] What they found was startling. Compared with placebo, newer sleep drugs (e.g. Ambien, Lunesta, and Sonata) produced only slight improvements in people's ability to fall asleep. These findings led the researchers to state, "...the drug effect and the placebo response were rather small and of questionable clinic importance...." **Essentially, this study should make us seriously consider the possibility that the risks of these drugs may greatly outweigh any benefit, especially when an equally effective and radically safer option like sleep transformation training exists.**

You can Probably Sleep without Pills

The information so far may be enough to lead you to avoid sleep medication. But what if you're already taking medication and are worried you won't be able to stop without a return of insomnia and its daytime consequences? If you approach the process of stopping sleep medication in the right way and with the appropriate support, there is a very high chance you can stop without any real negative consequences. More importantly, once you've stopped the medication there is a good chance you will actually sleep better than you are with the medication. There is a lot of research that supports the fact that people can successfully stop sleep medication. I'll talk about some of it here.

In 2002, a German sleep scientist named Goran Hajak and his associates completed a study on the effects of a single simple sleep transformation strategy on how people used sleep medication.[16] They studied 2690 people from 550 primary care clinics in Germany. Half of them received a prescription for the sleep medication Ambien to take a few nights per week as needed. The other half received the same prescription for Ambien and were also taught the Escape, Hang Out, Try Again process and a couple of other techniques (the same techniques I teach in the free SHARP Sleep Transformation video, which you can download for free at www.coloradoinsomniaclinic.com/sharpsleeptraining).

Guess what they found? Almost 70% of the people who were taught to use the sleep transformation techniques chose to use less medication.[16] What's more interesting is that they were just as satisfied with their treatment as people who did not receive the sleep transformation training, even though they used an average of 30% less medication. This is amazing to me (and to you too I hope)! **Simple changes in sleep behavior can help an overwhelming majority of people using Ambien take 30% less medication.** If you haven't watched it already, follow the link above to watch the SHARP sleep transformation video.

Another study provided people with insomnia who were using sleep medication with a series of small booklets about how to change their sleep without medication.[17] People in this study received the booklets along with supportive phone calls from a healthcare provider over a period of six weeks. Before they participated in the study patients were using sleep medication almost half the time. After following the recommendations in the booklets and having a few short conversations with a health provider, they were on average using medication only 7% of nights. **That means that after the study they were only using their sleep medication about twice per month.**

Now for the really impressive research. There have been several studies aimed at helping people get completely free of the most addictive sleep medications after years of using them every night. I'll talk about one of them here. Along with his colleagues, a Canadian sleep scientist named Charles Morin studied a group of adults with insomnia who had been using benzodiazepines (the most addictive type of sleep medication) for an average of more than 19 years.[18] Their goal was to help these individuals reduce or eliminate use of these medications using a process of supervised tapering in which medication was slowly reduced over a period of 10 weeks under the supervision of a physician. At the end of the 10 weeks more than 60% of the people in the study were completely drug free. This is absolutely remarkable! **The people who participated in this study had been using the equivalent of almost 10mg of diazepam (Valium) an average of 6.7 nights per week for almost 20 years and after only 10 weeks the majority of them were free of the medication.** What about those who were not able to totally stop using the medication? The majority also significantly reduced the amount of medication they were using to sleep. A couple more important points:

- 12 months after the study they were still using less or no sleep medication.

- When sleep transformation training was added to the supervised medication tapering process, 85% of participants were drug free at the end of the study.

- On average, participants were actually drug free in less than seven weeks, well before the 10 week study was completed.

- There was no increase in insomnia symptoms during or after reducing and eliminating the medication.

- Participants experienced very few withdrawal symptoms.

If these individuals, who were taking the most addictive type of sleep medication almost every night for more than a decade, can reduce or eliminate their sleep medication with no negative effects on their sleep, what is possible for you? Although there are many reasons why attempting to stop sleep medication may not be a good idea, it is always worth having a conversation with your medication prescriber.

You have to be your own advocate

Your medication prescriber will likely be overjoyed by your interest in learning how to stop using sleep medication. This is especially true if you come to him or her with a plan about how to do it and an alternative insomnia solution like sleep transformation training. Most primary care providers have a generally negative attitude toward prescribing sleep medication.[19] Additionally, they often have positive attitudes about reducing the use of sleep medication.[19] However, you will need to be your own advocate if you want help avoiding or stopping sleep medication use. I say this for several reasons.

First, the pharmaceutical industry has a powerful influence on prescribing patterns and habits in medical practice. The marketing guru Seth Godin gives us some insight into the reason for this influence, "In 2003 pharmaceutical companies spent more on marketing and sales than they did on research and development. When it comes time to invest, it's pretty clear that spreading the ideas behind the medicine is more important that inventing the medicine itself."[20] This seems true with reports from 2012 that the pharmaceutical company Purdue planned to spend $100 million over 12 months to promote the sleep drug Intermezzo, a special version of Ambien.[21] That's $100 million in marketing for one drug in a single year. Ultimately, this means that doctors (and we as consumers) are under a multi-billion dollar influence that teaches that drugs are safe and easy and the right and best thing to do.

Second, due to the marketing influence and many other reasons, medications hold a preferred status in our healthcare system. This means that it takes focused intentional effort on the part of you and your healthcare provider to successfully engage and follow through with non-medication alternatives like sleep transformation training. With that said, I'll finish this chapter by giving you an idea of how we approach the issue of helping you get free of sleep medication at The Insomnia Clinic.

The Insomnia Clinic Pathway: Sleep Medication Escape Plan

Earlier in the chapter I said that if you go about it the right way and you have the right support, you can probably get free of sleep medication. At The Insomnia Clinic, we approach the process of helping you get free of sleep medication in a specific way. There are three main steps:

1. Complete Guided Sleep Discovery – During this process we will determine all causes of your insomnia and create a plan for addressing them.

2. Radical Sleep Transformation – With your plan in hand, we work with you to strengthen your natural sleep systems, break down barriers, and overcome obstacles to natural sleep.

3. Sleep Medication Escape Plan – In collaboration with your medication prescriber we come up with a plan to slowly reduce and then eliminate your need for sleep medication using scientifically proven processes and techniques.

Each person's escape plan is tailored to their specific sleep medication and insomnia history. However these are some basic things to avoid when attempting to get free of sleep medication:

- Don't stop your medication suddenly unless directed to do so by your prescriber. You will almost certainly experience a return of significant insomnia symptoms unless you reduce the medication slowly.

- Don't try to stop your medication unless you have a plan for dealing with short-term insomnia symptoms that are likely to come up as you go through the process.

- Don't try to stop your sleep medication on your own. In some cases, stopping sleep medication can be dangerous and should always be supervised by a healthcare provider.

Summary

Sleep medications have an appropriate and necessary role within our healthcare system. However, they come with significant risks and in many cases are unnecessary. They are unnecessary for many individuals with insomnia because alternative solutions, like sleep transformation training, exist that are just as effective and less risky compared to medication. Despite the fact that excellent non-medication solutions are available, sleep medications remain the almost exclusive treatment for insomnia used by healthcare providers. Unfortunately, anytime someone starts sleep medication there is a high likelihood of becoming dependent. Fortunately, getting free from sleep medication is possible and there are clearly researched methods for doing so. We help motivated folks like you do it all the time at The Insomnia Clinic.

CHAPTER 18

HEALTHY SLEEP HABITS (SLEEP HYGIENE)

The activities you choose throughout the day and evening, what you put into your body (and when), and the bedroom environment you create can have a major influence on your sleep at night and how you feel during the day. In addition to everything else in this book, the following healthy sleep habits will further set the stage for a natural great night of sleep. There are six primary healthy sleep habits.

Caffeine

Murray Carpenter, the author of Caffeinated: How Our Daily Habit Helps, Hurts, and Hooks Us, calls caffeine, "America's drug of choice."[1,2] A tablespoon will kill you, but it's sold over the counter and can be found in many of the items you buy every day at the grocery store. It is regulated in drugs made by pharmaceutical companies, but has no limits when put in food. It is found everywhere: coffee, tea, soft drinks, chocolate, energy drinks, pain relievers, and supplements. And we use a lot of it. Worldwide we consume 20,000 Coca Cola soft drinks every SECOND![1] 1.7 billion every day. 54% of Americans drink coffee every day and average 3.1 9oz cups per day.3 We like caffeine so much we spend $40 billion per year on it.[3]

How much caffeine do you drink each day? How many cups of coffee, or sodas, or energy drinks? Be honest. When you say two cups do you mean two 8oz cups? Eight ounces is what is technically meant by a "cup" of coffee. Or do you mean two Starbucks Venti lattes (a total of 40 ounces)? Why do you drink it? Because it tastes good? Hopefully. You probably also drink it because it's a neuroenhancer. It makes you feel good. Through its effect on the brain, it makes you feel more alert, more focused, more energetic, and in a better mood. This is great when you want to be awake, but it's a problem if you would rather be sleeping.

One way caffeine makes us feel good is by blocking a chemical called adenosine. Adenosine builds up in the brain while you're awake. The longer you're awake the more you have and the more you have the sleepier you'll feel when bedtime comes. This chemical is also responsible for helping you fall asleep quickly, stay asleep, and sleep deeply.

Because of this, when it comes to sleep, the general recommendation is no caffeine within 6 hours of bedtime. But sleep scientist Chris Drake recently published a study that showed that caffeine even 6 hours before bed led to disrupted sleep.[4] So what are you to do?

Well, your sensitivity to caffeine is unique to you. You may say, "I'm still wired at bedtime if I have a sip of caffeine after 10am." If this is the case, then you should respect that and avoid caffeine after 10am. On the other hand you may say something like, "I drink a cup of coffee after dinner each night and I'm fine." Well, Dr. Drake's research also found that most people were not aware of the disruptive effects of caffeine on their sleep.[4] Caffeine may have effects on your sleep that are not obvious or don't make sense.

Whatever you believe about the effect of caffeine consumption on your sleep, if you're having trouble sleeping, the only way you can really know if caffeine is part of the problem is to stop using it for a little while. How do you do this? Let me assure you it can be done. The website www.caffeineinformer.com will show you a couple of ways to go about getting off of caffeine.[5] Just go to the site and search for "detox." They'll also give you a bunch of reasons (other than better sleep) why it's a good idea.

Alcohol

Alcohol is tricky. Like caffeine, its effects on sleep can be difficult to see.[6] What makes alcohol even trickier is that it works on the same part of the brain as sleeping pills. So, as you've probably noticed if you've ever drank alcohol around bedtime, it can actually cause sleepiness and make it easier to fall asleep. The problem is that although alcohol may help sleep at the beginning of the night, it changes sleep in a way that leads to more broken and restless sleep in the latter half of the night, when its effects begin to wear off. It can also cause early morning awakenings with an inability to return to sleep.

You may enjoy a drink or two in the evenings and feel that this has little or no effect on your sleep. You may be right but the negative effects of alcohol on sleep are often subtle and hard to pin down to the couple of drinks you had around dinner time.

You may find yourself using alcohol to help make it easier to get to sleep or return to sleep. Drinking alcohol is one of the most common ways that that individuals with insomnia "self-medicate."[7] This is problematic as there are some estimates that suggest some cases of alcohol dependence and abuse may be caused by using alcohol in an effort to overcome insomnia.[8,9] Additionally, over time, frequent use of alcohol can actually have reverse effects, leading to more difficulty getting to sleep rather than less.[6]

For these reasons, it is a good idea to avoid drinking alcohol in the evenings. Like caffeine, the only real way to know if alcohol is having an effect on your sleep pattern is to stop using it for a while.

Food

What have you heard about eating before bedtime? Are you supposed to have a snack before bed? Are you not supposed to eat anything after 9 pm (remember the movie Gremlins?)? Well this is a bit of a double edged sword.

Eat too much and your body may be trying to digest when you're trying to sleep and you may have more acid reflux or GERD (Gastroesophageal Reflux Disease), which can disrupt sleep. In fact, my mentor and friend Bill Orr is one of the pioneers of research on what happens when you have GERD during the night. It's not pretty. When you're sleeping, it takes more acid sitting in your esophagus for a longer period of time before you will get a feeling of heartburn. This means you could be having GERD every night and not know that it is the cause of poor quality sleep.

On the other hand, you don't want to go to bed hungry. How are you supposed to sleep when your stomach is growling or aching? Ok. Here is how to handle it. First, avoid meals within 2 or 3 hours before bedtime. Second, a light snack within the hour before bed may actually help you feel sleepier.

Now that you have those clear recommendations, you probably have another question. What should I eat for a snack? There are plenty of recommendations out there. I don't think there is any right snack but there are some people who claim this type of food or that type of food are "sleep superfoods." Eating Well.com lists nine foods to help sleep:[10]

- Fish (especially salmon) gives you vitamin B6, which your body can use to make melatonin, a hormone connected to sleep.

- Bananas, fortified cereals, and chickpeas are also good sources of B6.

- Jasmine rice, which has a higher glycemic index than regular long-grain rice, might help you fall asleep faster.

- People who have insomnia sleep better when drinking a cup of Tart Cherry juice twice a day. It has lots of melatonin.

- Yogurt, which is high in calcium, may help sleep in folks with low calcium.

- Green leafy vegetables like Kale and collards have a lot of calcium too.

- Whole grains like bulgur barley contain lots of magnesium that may also help sleep.

If these suggestions aren't enough for you, I typed "Bedtime Snacks" into Google and came up with 903,000 results in 0.32 seconds. I'm sure you can find some interesting ideas to try.

Comfortable Environment

How would you describe your bed? Comfy and cozy? Like sleeping on a bed of nails? How would you describe your bedroom? A calming oasis amidst the frenzied chaos of day-to-day living? A cave with carpet? Or maybe a second office? Comfort is important. In order to let go into blissful sleep we need to have a sense of safety and comfort. This means you need to have a comfortable bed. You don't necessarily need to go out and spend thousands on a new bed, but if your mattress looks more like a hammock it's time for a change. The general recommendation is to replace your mattress every 8-10 years. While you're at it, it may be a good idea to have some comfortable pillows and blankies as well. This also means you should probably take the time to make your bedroom an enjoyable place to be. Maybe some nice lighting, some curtains, and a lavender candle or two. Make some effort to make your bedroom a place you can look forward to going at the end of the day.

While we're talking about comfort, we also need to talk about light, noise, and temperature. Our bodies were designed to be awake in the daylight and asleep in the dark. So it's important to minimize the amount of light in the bedroom when you're trying to sleep. Basically, you want to have enough light so nobody gets injured making their way to the bathroom in the middle of the night. Also, in most cases it's a good idea to limit the amount of natural light that comes into the bedroom in the mornings, as morning light can be a signal for your brain that it's time to start the day.

It probably goes without saying, a quiet environment is ideal for sleep. But, getting your environment to cooperate can be difficult. Neighbor's dogs and snoring spouses are the most common sources of unwanted nighttime noise. (Hint - you're not supposed to sleep when the person you love is choking in the bed right next to you. They should talk to their doc-tor. There are many solutions to these noises but most of them aren't very kind.)

So what are you to do? There are two main options that you have 100% control over: earplugs and white noise. You can find 10 different kinds of earplugs at your local drugstore. They may feel a bit uncomfortable the first few days but once you get used to them they may be a great solution. If you're not into earplugs then consider getting something that generates white noise. You might use a fan or humidifier. There are also white noise machines that generate a variety of sounds like waterfalls or rainforests. Be careful with these however. Any sounds that are not constant and meaningless are not technically white noise and have the potential to dis-rupt sleep. TV and audiobooks are definitely not considered white noise. Unless you're a parent or caregiver who needs to keep an ear out during the night, these can be quite helpful.

Now, what about temperature? There is no "right" temperature for sleep but in general you can think that sleep loves the cold. Also, it is usually easier to make the bedroom cold and control your own temperature with sheets and blankets, than to make the room warm and try figure out how to keep yourself cool. With this in mind, you will probably find that a cool bedroom supports a better night's sleep.

Tobacco is a Stimulant

What about nicotine? Is it okay to have a smoke right before bed? What about when you wake up during the night? The bottom line is that whether it is from cigarettes, chewing tobacco, patches or gum, nicotine is a stim-ulant.[11] Because of this, nicotine makes it take longer to fall asleep and reduces deep sleep.

Given these facts, the best option is to quit. The initial time after quitting can be temporarily challenging. But, even if you're a long-term smoker who feels that having a cigarette calms you down, you will most likely find that your sleep improves if you quit. With that said, I understand that quit-ting tobacco is easier said than done. I actually quit smoking about 15 years ago, so I know how difficult it can be. If you're not able to quit, there are some things you can do to minimize the effect of nicotine on your sleep.

First, reduce the total amount of nicotine you use each day as much as you are able. Going a little longer than usual between each chew or cigarette, or choosing to skip one every now and then can sometimes be easy ways to use less. Second, plan to avoid nicotine near bedtime and during middle of night awakenings. The less nicotine you have in your system, the more likely you will be to sleep deeply.

Exercise

Do you ever try to exhaust yourself by exercising hard for a long time in the hopes of making yourself sleepy? How has that worked for you? If you're like most people, not very well. The relationship between exercise and sleep is not exactly clear. Although there is at least one study that says an hour of moderate exercise 4-5 hours before bed can reduce bedtime anxiety and help you fall asleep faster, in general it is unlikely that exercise today will help you sleep better tonight.[12-13]

However, individuals who exercise regularly seem to sleep better than those who don't. So, if you are already fairly fit and exercise regularly, then increasing your exercise probably won't help you much. Give yourself a pat on the back for already following this healthy sleep habit. If you're not exercising regularly, then changing this habit may have a big impact on your sleep. This appears especially true for older adults and individuals who have anxiety in addition to insomnia.

Whatever category you're in, there is one clear rule about exercise for healthy sleep. No moderate to high intensity exercise within 2-3 hours of bedtime. Think about it. When you exercise intensely your body gets activated and your body temperature increases. If you activate your body then you have to give it a chance to deactivate in order to be ready for sleep. For most of us that takes a while.

Summary

There are six primary healthy sleep habits:

- Limit caffeine within 6 hours of bedtime

- Make your bed and bedroom as comfortable as possible

- Reduce or eliminate nicotine, especially before bed and during the night

- Limit alcohol use within 2-3 hours of bedtime

- Eat a light snack around bedtime, but avoid meals within 2-3 hours of going to bed

- Exercise regularly, but not within 2-3 hours of bedtime

Any one of these can make a difference for you. You know the ones you're already doing well and you know the ones you need to focus on changing. The more of them you follow, the more likely you are to see a difference in your ability to fall asleep, sleep deeply, wake up less, sleep longer, and feel more rested.

You may be thinking, "I've heard all these before." If so, you may be tempted to ignore them. Just because you've heard them before doesn't mean they're not useful. Don't fall into that trap. **These kinds of changes are recommended so often because they are so simple and so important.** Or, you may be thinking, "I've tried that, it doesn't work for me." Keep in mind that consistency is the key to success. In order to see the real benefit of these kinds of changes you probably need to follow them for at least two weeks. Maybe more. If you're serious about sleeping better then I encourage you to commit to making as many of these changes as you're able for at least two weeks.

Things like caffeine, nicotine, alcohol, food, exercise, and our sleep environment have a real impact on sleep and they impact sleep in ways that may not be obvious. This means that making the kinds of changes I've suggested offers a real opportunity for better sleep. Which one will you begin to change today? Pick one and begin your journey toward better sleep.

BIBLIOGRAPHY

Chapter 1 - Introduction

1. Morin C, Vallières A, Guay B, Ivers H, Savard J, Mérette C, et al. Cognitive behavioral therapy, singly and combined with medication, for persistent insomnia: a randomized controlled trial. JAMA 2009;301:2005-2015.

2. Individuals certified in behavioral sleep medicine by the American Board of Sleep Medicine as of February 2015: http://www.absm.org/bsmspecialists.aspx

3. Glidewell R, Renn B, Roby E, Orr W. Predictors and patterns of insomnia symptoms in OSA before and after PAP therapy. Sleep Medicine 2014;15:899-905.

4. Glidewell R, Roby E, Orr W. Is insomnia an independent predictor of obstructive sleep apnea? J Am Board Fam Med 2012;25:104-110.

5. Glidewell R, Moorcroft W, Lee-Chiong Jr. T. Comorbid insomnia: Reciprocal relationships and medication management. Sleep Medicine Clinics 2010;5:627-646.

6. http://www.npr.org/blogs/health/2014/01/27/265254533/how-parents-and-the-internet-transformed-clubfoot-treatment

7. Espie C (2014). Presentation at the annual meeting of the Associated Professional Sleep Societies, Minneapolis, MN.

8. NIH state of the science conference statement on manifestations and management of chronic insomnia in adults. J Clin Sleep Med 2005;1:412-421.

Chapter 2 - My Story Part I: Insomniac to Insomnia Expert

1. Glidewell R. The importance of sleep disturbance on physical and mental health: A proposal for increased clinic attention. Colorado School of Professional Psychology 2003.

2. Glidewell R. Considering Sleep Part I: Implications of sleep disturbance for clinic practice. Colorado School of Professional Psychology 2004.

3. Glidewell R. Glidewell Rapid Sleep Screen: A structured interview for identifying and managing sleep disturbance. Doctoral Dissertation. Colorado School of Professional Psychology 2006. http://gradworks.umi.com/32/96/3296913.html

4. Glidewell R, Renn B, Roby E, Orr W. Predictors and patterns of insomnia symptoms in OSA before and after PAP therapy. Sleep Medicine 2014;15:899-905.

5. Glidewell R. Comorbid insomnia and sleep disordered breathing. Curr Treat Options Neurol. 2013: DOI 10.1007/s11940-013-0259-0.

6. Glidewell R, Roby E, Orr W. Is insomnia an independent predictor of obstructive sleep apnea? J Am Board Fam Med 2012;25(1):104-110.

7. Glidewell R, Moorcroft W, Lee-Chiong Jr. T. Comorbid insomnia: Reciprocal relationships and medication management. Sleep Medicine Clinics 2010;5:627-646.

8. Glidewell R, Botts E, Orr W. Insomnia and anxiety: Diagnostic and management implications of complex interactions. Sleep Medicine Clinics 2015;10:93-99.

Chapter 3 – My Story Part II: Birth of the Sleep Health Revolution

1. Mindell J, Bartle A, Wahab N, Ahn Y, Ramamurthy M, Huong H. Sleep education in medical school curriculum: A glimpse across countries. Sleep Medicine 2011;12:928-931.

2. Rosen R, Zozula R. Education and training in the field of sleep medicine. Current Opinion in Pulmonary Medicine 2000;6:512-518.

3. Godin S. All Marketers are Liars. New York 2003: Penguin.

4. http://www.skainfo.com/health_care_market_reports/2012_promotional_spending.pdf

5. http://www.pewtrusts.org/en/research-and-analysis/factsheets/2013/11/11/persuading-the-prescribers-pharmaceutical-industry-marketing-and-its-influence-on-physicians-and-patients

Chapter 4 - LAW #1: Sleep is Critically Essential

1. Cheung J, Bartlett D, Armour C. The insomnia patient perspective: A narrative review. Behavioral Sleep Medicine 2013;5:369-389.

2. http://www.thefiscaltimes.com/Articles/2013/07/16/How-a-Bad-Nights-Sleep-Can-Derail-Your-Career

3. Daley M, Morin C, LeBlanc M, Gregoire J, Savard J. The economic burden of insomnia: Direct and indirect costs for individuals with insomnia syndrome, insomnia symptoms, and good sleepers. SLEEP 2009;32:55-64.

4. Sarsour K, Kalsekar A, Swindle R, Foley K, Walsh J. The association between insomnia severity and healthcare productivity costs in a health plan sample. SLEEP 2011;34:443-450.

5. Leger D, Massuel M, Metlaine A, SISYPHE Study Group. Profes-
    sional correlates of insomnia. SLEEP 2006;29:171-178.

6. http://www.today.com/id/43357508/ns/today-today_health/t/
    sleepy-wife-may-take-it-out-hubby/#.UrD1FfRDt8E

7. http://blog.doctoroz.com/oz-experts/could-insomnia-pose-a-
    cancer-risk

Chapter 5 - LAW #2: Insomnia Has Many Causes

1. Lichstein K, Riedel B, Lester K, Aguillard N. Occult sleep apnea in a
    recruited sample of older adults with insomnia. J Clin Consulting
    Psychology 1999;67:405-410.

Chapter 6 – LAW #3: Insomnia has a Life of Its Own

1. Lichstein K, Wilson N, Johnson C. Psychological treatment of sec-
    ondary insomnia. Psychology and Aging 2000;15:232-240.

2. Smith M, Haythornthwaite J. How do sleep disturbance and
    chronic pain interrelate? Insights from the longitudinal and cogni-
    tive-behavioral clinical trials literature. Sleep Med Rev 2004;8:119-
    132.

3. Currie S, Wilson K, Pontefract A, deLaplante L. Cognitive behavioral
    treatment of insomnia secondary to chronic pain. J Clin Consulting
    Psychology 2000;68:407-416.

4. Vitiello M, Rybarczyk B, Von Korff M, Stepanski E. Cognitive behav-
    ioral therapy for insomnia improves sleep and decreases pain in
    older adults with co-morbid Insomnia and osteoarthritis. Sleep
    Med 2009;5:355-362.

5. Manber R, Chambers A. Insomnia and depression: A multifaceted
    interplay. Current Psychiatry Reports 2009;11:437-442.

6. Savard J, Simard S, Ivers H, Morin C. Randomized study on the ef-
    ficacy of cognitive-behavioral therapy for insomnia secondary to

breast cancer, part 1: Sleep and psychological effects. J Clin Oncol 2005;23:6083-6096.

7. Glidewell R, Botts E, Orr W. Insomnia and anxiety: Diagnostic and management implications of complex interactions. Sleep Medicine Clinics 2015;10:93-99.

8. Glidewell R. Comorbid insomnia and sleep disordered breathing. Curr Treat Options Neurol. 2013: DOI 10.1007/s11940-013-0259-0.

9. Glidewell R, Renn B, Roby E, Orr W. Predictors and patterns of insomnia symptoms in OSA before and after PAP therapy. Sleep Medicine 2014;15:899-905.

10. Glidewell R, Moorcroft W, Lee-Chiong Jr. T. Comorbid insomnia: Reciprocal relationships and medication management. Sleep Medicine Clinics 2010;5:627-646.

11. Rybarczyk B, Lopez M, Schelble K, Stepanski E. Home-based video CBT for comorbid geriatric insomnia: A pilot study using secondary data analysis. Behavioral Sleep Medicine 2005;3:158-175.

12. Espie C (2014). Presentation at the annual meeting of the Associated Professional Sleep Societies, Minneapolis, MN.

Chapter 9 - LAW #6: Insomnia is a Programming Problem

1. Morin C. Psychological and behavioral treatments for insomnia I: Approaches and efficacy. In M. Kryger, T. Roth, and W. Dement (Eds.) *Principles and practice of sleep medicine* (5th Ed.; pp. 866-882). St. Louis, MO 2011: Elsevier-Saunders.

2. Glidewell RN, Renn BN, Roby E, Orr WC. Predictors and patterns of insomnia symptoms in OSA before and after PAP therapy. Sleep Medicine 2014;15:899-905.

Chapter 10 - LAW #7: Insomnia is a Mind Problem

1. Morin C, Espie C. Insomnia: A clinical guide to assessment and treatment. New York 2003: Kluwer Academic/Plenum Publishers.

2. Jordana Cooperberg, MA, The Causes of Insomnia, PAH Behavioral Health Clinic Newsletter, April 2011: http://www.med.upenn.edu/psychotherapy/user_documents/CausesofInsomnia.

3. Dysfunctional Beliefs and Attitudes About Sleep (DBAS) Scale. Morin C. Insomnia: Psychological assessment and management. New York 1993: The Guilford Press. You can download it here: http://www.fss.ulaval.ca/cms_recherche/upload/chaire_sommeil/fichiers/dysfunctional_beliefs_and_attitudes_about_sleep_30_items.pdf

Chapter 13 - LAW #10: Insomnia is a Stress problem

1. http://www.psychwiki.com/wiki/Zeigarnik_Effect

2. Goleman D. Social intelligence: The new science of human relationships. New York 2006: Bantam Books.

3. http://content.time.com/time/covers/0,16641,20140203,00.html

4. Gross C, Kreitzer M, Reilly-Spong M, Wall M, Winbush N, Patterson R, et al. Mindfulness-based stress reduction vs pharmacotherapy for primary chronic insomnia: A pilot randomized controlled clinical trial. Explore (NY) 2011;7:76-87.

5. Ong J, Shapiro S, Manber R. Combining mindfulness meditation with cognitive-behavior therapy for insomnia: A treatment-development study. Behavior Therapy 2008;39:171-182.

6. Ong J, Shapiro S, Manber R. Mindfulness meditation and cognitive behavioral therapy for insomnia: A naturalistic 12-month follow-up. Explore 2009;5:30-36.

Chapter 17 – The Truth about Sleep Medication

1. Morin C, LeBlanc M, Belanger L, Ivers H, Merette C, Savard J. Prevalence of insomnia and its treatment in Canada. Can J Psychiatry 2011;56:540-548.

2. NIH state of the science conference statement on manifestations and management of chronic insomnia in adults. J Clin Sleep Med 2005;1:412-421.

3. Morin C, Vallières A, Guay B, Ivers H, Savard J, Mérette C, et al. Cognitive behavioral therapy, singly and combined with medication, for persistent insomnia: a randomized controlled trial. JAMA 2009;301:2005-2015.

4. Lichstein K, Wilson N, Johnson C. Psychological treatment of secondary insomnia. Psychology and Aging 2000;15:232-240.

5. Smith M, Haythornthwaite J. How do sleep disturbance and chronic pain interrelate? Insights from the longitudinal and cognitive-behavioral clinical trials literature. Sleep Med Rev 2004;8:119-132.

6. Currie S, Wilson K, Pontefract A, deLaplante L. Cognitive behavioral treatment of insomnia secondary to chronic pain. J Clin Consulting Psychology 2000;68:407-416.

7. Vitiello M, Rybarczyk B, Von Korff M, Stepanski E. Cognitive behavioral therapy for insomnia improves sleep and decreases pain in older adults with co-morbid insomnia and osteoarthritis. Sleep Med 2009;5:355-362.

8. Manber R, Chambers A. Insomnia and depression: A multifaceted interplay. Current Psychiatry Reports 2009;11:437-442.

9. Savard J, Simard S, Ivers H, Morin C. Randomized study on the efficacy of cognitive-behavioral therapy for insomnia secondary to breast cancer, part 1: Sleep and psychological effects. J Clin Oncol 2005;23:6083-6096.

10. Glidewell R, Botts E, Orr W. Insomnia and anxiety: Diagnostic and management implications of complex interactions. Sleep Medicine Clinics 2015;10:93-99.

11. Glidewell RN. Comorbid insomnia and sleep disordered breathing. Curr Treat Options Neurol. 2013: DOI 10.1007/s11940-013-0259-0.

12. Glidewell R, Moorcroft W, Lee-Chiong Jr. T. Comorbid insomnia: Reciprocal relationships and medication management. Sleep Medicine Clinics 2010;5(4):627-646.

13. Rybarczyk B, Lopez M, Schelble K, Stepanski E. Home-based video CBT for comorbid geriatric insomnia: A pilot study using secondary data analysis. Behavioral Sleep Medicine 2005;3:158-175.

14. Smith M, Perlis M, Park A, Smith M, Pennington J, Giles D, et al., Comparative meta-analysis of pharmacotherapy and behavior therapy for persistent insomnia. Am J Psychiatry 2002;159:5-11.

15. Hueda-Medina T, Kirsch I, Middlemass J, Klonizakis M, Siriwardena A. Effectiveness of non-benzodiazepine hypnotics in treatment of adult insomnia: Meta-analysis of data submitted to the food and drug administration. BMJ 2012;345; e8343 doi: 10.1136/bmj.e8343.

16. Hajak G, Bandelow B, Zulley J, Pittrow D. "As Needed" pharmacotherapy combined with stimulus control treatment in chronic insomnia: Assessment of a novel intervention strategy in a primary care setting. Ann Clin Psychiatry 2002;14:1-7.

17. Mimeault V, Morin C. Self-help treatment for insomnia: Bibliotherapy with and without professional guidance. JCCP 1999;67:511-519.

18. Morin C, Bastien C, Guay B, Radouco-Thomas M, Leblanc J, Vallieres A. Randomized clinical trial of supervised tapering and cognitive behavior therapy to facilitate benzodiazepine discontinuation in older adults with chronic insomnia. Am J Psychiatry 2004;161:332-342.

19. Siriwardena A, Apekey T, Tilling M, Dyas J, Middleton H, Orner R. General practitioners' preferences for managing insomnia and opportunities for reducing hypnotic prescribing. Journal of Evaluation in Clinical Practice 2010;16:731-737.

20. Godin S. All Marketers are Liars. New York 2003: Penguin.

21. http://adage.com/article/news/intermezzo-rouses-drug-category-100-million-push/234014/

Chapter 18 - Healthy Sleep Habits (Sleep Hygiene)

1. Carpenter M. Caffeinated: How Our Daily Habit Helps, Hurts, and Hooks Us. New York 2014. Hudson Street Press.

2. https://soundcloud.com/nationalgeographicradio/caffeine-americas-drug-of

3. http://www.hsph.harvard.edu/news/multimedia-article/facts/

4. Drake C, Roehrs T, Shambroom J, Roth T. Caffeine effects on sleep taken 0, 3, or 6 hours before going to bed. J Clin Sleep Med 2013;9:1195-1200.

5. http://www.caffeineinformer.com/my-caffeine-detox

6. Brower K. Alcohol's effects on sleep in alcoholics. Alcohol Research and Health 2001;25:110-125.

7. Johnson E, Roehrs T, Roth T, and Breslau N. Epidemiology of alcohol and medication as aids to sleep in early adulthood. SLEEP 1998;21:178-186.

8. Stoller M. Economic effects of insomnia. Clinical therapeutics 1994;16:873-897.

9. Ford D, Kamerow D. Epidemiologic study of sleep disturbances and psychiatric disorders: An opportunity for prevention. JAMA 1989;262:1479-1484.

10. http://www.eatingwell.com/nutrition_health/ nutrition_news_information/9_foods_to_help_you_sleep

11. Jaehne A, Loessl B, Barkai Z, Riemann D, Hornyak. Effects of nicotine on sleep during consumption, withdrawal, and replacement therapy. Sleep Med Rev 2009;13:363-377.

12. Passos G, Poyares D, Santana M, Garbuio S, Tufik S, Mello M. Effect of acute physical exercise on patients with chronic primary insomnia. J Clin Sleep Med 2010;6:270-275.

13. Passos G, Poyares D, Santana M, D'Aurea C, Youngstedt S, Tufik S, et al. Effects of moderate aerobic exercise training on chronic primary insomnia. Sleep Med 2011;12:1018-1027.

ABOUT THE AUTHOR

ROBERT N. GLIDEWELL, PSYD, CBSM

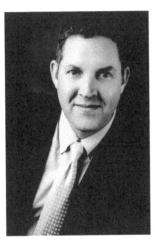

Dr. Glidewell is founder of The Insomnia Clinic and a member of the Sleep Health Revolution. He is one of fewer than 200 psychologists worldwide to be awarded certification in Behavioral Sleep Medicine by the American Board of Sleep Medicine. He has extensive advanced training in the diagnosis and treatment of sleep disorders to include training at the Duke University Insomnia and Sleep Research Program. He has evaluated and treated hundreds of individuals with chronic and complex insomnia, dependence on sleeping pills, fatigue, excessive daytime sleepiness, and a range of other sleep and associated problems. He has published original research, case studies, and reviews in the Journal of Clinical Sleep Medicine, the Journal of the American Board of Family Medicine, Sleep Medicine Clinics, Current Treatment Options in Neurology, and the journal Sleep Medicine. He is also the author of numerous scientific abstracts related to his original research on topics including the assessment of sleep disorders and the interactions between sleep apnea, insomnia, and use of CPAP therapies. He moved to Colorado Springs, Colorado in 1995 during his service in the United States Air Force. He continues to live in Colorado Springs with his wife and two children. Learn more about Dr. Glidewell, The Insomnia Clinic, and the Sleep Health Revolution at www.coloradoinsomniaclinic.com.